201 S‹
High-Performance
Optometric Practice

Bob Levoy

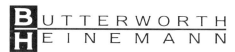

An Imprint of Elsevier Science

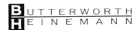
An Imprint of Elsevier Science

225 Wildwood Avenue
Woburn, MA 01801

ISBN 0-7506-7325-7

Copyright © 2002, Elsevier Science. All rights reserved.

Notice

Optometry is an ever-changing field. Standard safety precautions must be followed, but as new research and clinical experience broaden our knowledge, changes in treatment and drug therapy may become necessary or appropriate. Readers are advised to check the most current product information provided by the manufacturer of each drug to be administered to verify the recommended dose, the method and duration of administration, and contraindications. It is the responsibility of the treating physician, relying on experience and knowledge of the patient, to determine dosages and the best treatment for each individual patient. Neither the Publisher nor the author assume any liability for any injury and/or damage to persons or property arising from this publication.

The Publisher

Editorial Staff Acknowledgments:

Publishing Director: Linda Duncan
Managing Editor: Christie M. Hart
Project Manager: Mary Stermel

Library of Congress Cataloging-in-Publication Data

Levoy, Robert P.
   201 secrets of a high performance optometric practice / Bob Levoy.
     p. cm.
   ISBN 0-7506-7325-7
    1. Optometry--Practice. I. Title: Two hundred one secrets of a high performance optometric practice. II. Title.

RE959.3 .L48 2003
617.7'5'068--dc21

2002026152

SSC/MVY

Printed in the United States of America
Last digit is the print number: 9 8 7 6 5 4 3 2

To Lynn and Brett, with much love

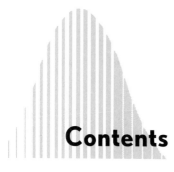

Contents

Chapter 2: Long-Range, Strategic Planning   33

Chapter 3: Major Opportunities for Revenue Enhancement and Practice Growth   41

Chapter 4: Secrets of Savvy Networking 67

Chapter 5: Getting to "Yes" 87

Chapter 6: Patient Expectations, Satisfaction, and Loyalty   **105**

Chapter 10: Brass Tacks of Personnel Management   177

Chapter 11: How to Keep Staff Motivation in High Gear   199

Chapter 12: Secrets of Stress Management   219

Special Thanks

'm indebted to many people for their invaluable help with the development of this book.

I'll start with countless optometrists who, with their staffs, have attended my seminars, provided feedback; allowed me to visit their practices, "pick their brains," talk with their patients; and shared their secrets of a high-performance practice.

There have been innumerable others in a wide range of professions whose "hard-learned lessons" appear throughout the pages of this book.

In the course of researching this book, there have been many people who took time from their busy schedules to provide vital information and valuable insights. These include Drs. Craig Andrews, Irving Bennett, Dan Bintz, Willard Bleything, Marc Bloomenstein, Drew Brooks, Charles Brownlow, Brian Chou, Bobby Christensen, Jason Clopton, Vic Connors, Noah Eger, Arthur Epstein, Neil Gailmard, Gary Gerber, Stuart Gindoff, Paul Harris, Alan Homestead, Erwin Jay, Jim Leadingham, Bernard Leibman, Malcolm McCannel, Ron Melton, Beverly Miller, Pamela Miller, Byron Newman, Gary Osias, Gregg Ossip, Roger Pabst, Thomas Porter, Leonard Press, Jack Runninger, Peter Shaw-McMinn, Gray Sass, Morris Sheffer, Robert Simmons, David Sullins, Andrea Thau, Nancy Torgerson, Jeffrey Weaver, Robert Wilson, and Joel Zaba. Other key people include Arnold Abramowitz, Christine Bauder, Joe Brueni, Carol Glick, Judith DuChateau, Linda Hines, Larisa Hubbs, Will Kuhlman, Thomas Lecoq, Dan Lex, Jeff Moss, John Murphy, Karen Pirino, Mike Smith, and Susan Thomas.

I am indebted also to Karen Oberheim, former medical publisher at Butterworth–Heinemann, for her support of this project from the moment she learned of it; Christie M. Hart, Managing Editor at Elsevier Science, and Brooke Begin, Production Editor, for skillfully steering the book through editing and production. I'd also like to thank an old friend,

Bob Williams, Executive Director of the Optometric Extension Program, for his encouragement and enthusiasm from the very start. And last, my most special thanks is to my wife, Martha, for her unending patience and support and her unerring copyediting and judgment.

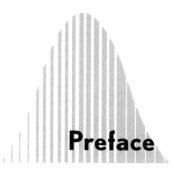

Preface

High-Performance Optometric Practice

There are many definitions of high performance. The Malcolm Baldrige National Quality Award Program created by Congress in 1987 defines it as, "Work approaches used to systematically pursue ever higher levels of overall organizational and individual performance including quality, productivity, innovation rate, and cycle time performance."[1]

The term, *high-performance optometric practice*, as used in this book, refers to *above-average levels of*:

Patient satisfaction
Patient loyalty
Employee motivation
Referrals
Profitability

Teamwork
Practice growth
Productivity
Patient acceptance
Professional prestige

Above-average achievement in these categories places high-performance optometric practices at the upper end (shaded portion) of the familiar *bell-shaped curve* shown throughout this book. This curve, the most widely used model in statistics, depicts a frequency distribution with the percent of optometric practices shown on the vertical ordinate (from low to high) and the magnitude of each achievement depicted on the horizontal ordinate (from below average on the left to above average on the right).

What does this select group of high-performance optometric practices have in common to have attained these above-average achievements? The answer in simplest terms is that *they have the right people, in the right jobs, doing the right things, at the right time.*

Obviously, there's more to the story—all of which unfolds in this book.

REAL PRACTICES, REAL SOLUTIONS

In the course of my career, I've had the privilege of conducting more than 2,500 seminars for a wide range of businesses and professional groups throughout North America and overseas. As part of the market research for these programs, I've visited countless professional practices, not only in optometry, but also in medicine, dentistry, podiatry, physical therapy, veterinary medicine, accounting, and law, among others. It has enabled me to meet hundreds of high-performance practitioners in each of these professions and ask them such questions as the following:

- What makes your practice so successful?
- What are you doing differently than others to account for your success?
- What are the secrets of hiring top-notch employees, and how do you keep them motivated?
- What have been your toughest management problems, and how did you solve them?
- What do you wish you had done differently?
- What lessons did you learn that may help others avoid costly mistakes?

Their answers became the foundation of this book.

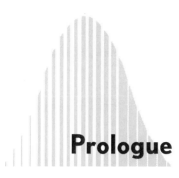

Prologue

Practice Management Revolution

The day before conducting a seminar in Vancouver, BC, Canada for the Continuing Legal Education Society of British Columbia, I met with Paul Beckman, a prominent attorney in Vancouver. He told me how crowded and competitive the law profession had become in his province. There were fewer clients because of mergers, acquisitions, and in-house counsels. There was an increase in non-lawyers who now offer services that were once the province of lawyers. "We used to walk through the forest," he said, "and the nuts would just fall out of the trees. That's not happening today."

I thought of those words as I started this book. They struck me as an apt metaphor for what is also happening in optometry.

A practice management revolution has taken place. What used to be the simple formula for success: *ability, affability, and availability*—the three As, as they were called—is, today, woefully inadequate. To achieve success in today's environment, much more is needed. Among the reasons is more competition, much of it cutthroat; increasing penetration of managed care; declining reimbursement rates by third-party payers; rising overheads; changing demographics; and a new breed of patient who is better informed, more cynical and demanding, more cost conscious, and less loyal than ever.

REALITY CHECK

What you've done to get your practice where it is today is no longer adequate to keep it there.

Many practice management ideas of the past are now ineffective, if not counter-productive. What's needed is new thinking, new strategies, and skills to attract and retain patients, generate referrals, and achieve a high-performance optometric practice.

1

Give Your Practice a Competitive Advantage

Business guru Tom Peters said at a recent seminar that private practice owners must create something special to stand out in a world of surpluses. He noted that we live in a surplus society, which is a society full of similar companies with similar ideas, employing similar people with similar educational backgrounds and experiences, and producing similar things, with similar quality and similar prices.[1]

Peters was talking to physical therapists, but his description of a surplus, commoditized society is equally true for optometrists.

1 Avoid the "commodity trap"

A *commodity* is a product in which brands are not perceived to be very different from one another. Examples are sugar, salt, and cotton: People think they're all the same, and in many cases just look for which is cheapest.

Unfortunately, there are many patients who think an eye examination is also a "commodity"—that is, *standard in all respects*, regardless of who does it. To their way of thinking, an examination is an examination. A prescription is a prescription.

"Market forces are turning contact lenses into a commodity," says Kenneth A. Lebow, O.D., Virginia Beach, VA.[2]

It's the same story for laser-assisted in situ keratomileusis (LASIK), which many patients have come to see as a commodity, writes Jeffrey S. Eisenberg, Senior Editor, *Review of Optometry*.[3]

The best way, in fact, the *only* way to avoid the commodity trap is to *differentiate* your practice. It means having something about your practice that sets it apart from others in what professor Michael Porter of Harvard University calls "substantial and sustainable ways." That is what gives your practice a *competitive advantage*. Positions it at the high end of the bell-shaped curve. Makes it *impervious* to competition and "price comparisons."

REALITY CHECK

If what you are doing in your practice is no better or no different (or *perceived* to be no better or different) than what's being done in offices that charge less, then what incentive do patients have to be in your practice? As William James observed, "A difference that makes no difference—is not a difference."

The following are among the many varied ways that high-performance optometrists have differentiated their practices: Think of them as a menu of possibilities.

2 A commitment to excellence

"There is considerable evidence," William Andres, former chairman of the Dayton-Hudson Corporation told the Harvard Business School Marketing Club, "that the very best businesses concentrate almost single-mindedly on serving the customer. Pleasing customers," he said, "is an *obsession*. Service is an *obsession*. Quality is an *obsession*. Dependability is an *obsession*. Attention to detail is an *obsession*."

His advice is dead-on for any service-driven business, optometry included.

The word *obsession* is the key. It implies not just a "lip service" promise to do these things, but rather a no-excuse, unswerving *commitment* to quality, service, dependability, and attention to detail.

For many practices, *growth* is king. For high-performance optometric practices, *excellence* is king.

"First be *best*, then be *first*." These words, spoken by Grant Tinker when he became chairman of NBC, articulated the philosophy that guided the network to its number one position during his tenure.

HARD-LEARNED LESSON

In today's highly competitive environment, good enough is simply not good enough.

---

3 Develop a niche practice

The name of the practice says it all: Alderwood Vision Therapy Center in Lynnwood, Washington. "I do evaluations and vision therapy—no dispensing, no glasses, no contact lenses," says Nancy G. Torgerson, O.D., F.C.O.V.D., current president of the College of Optometrists in Vision Development, "and we *love* what we do."

At one time, the *mass market* was every optometrist's target population. However, the best strategy today is "niche marketing." This means targeting a specific population of patients, identifying their needs, and then addressing those needs more competently than anyone else does.

"If you're the only practice in the community," says Ken Gibson, O.D., Appleton, WI, "you can be all things to all people. But, if you're in an urban area or in a town with more than two or three other optometrists, you need to set yourself apart—with a specialty practice."[4]

Also, by focusing on a specific segment of the population, you're more likely to know what those patients want and provide them with a higher level of satisfaction than you are providing—trying to be all things to all people.

ANOTHER MAJOR BENEFIT

When a practice is truly tailored to a particular segment of the population, patients tend to be less price sensitive.

There are more opportunities for specialty practice in optometry than ever. You simply need to find a niche to your liking (and for which there is a need in your community), obtain the needed training, and then get the word out. Among the many possibilities are the following:

Pediatrics
Learning-related visual problems
Orthokeratology
Therapeutics
Specialized contact lenses
Low vision

Co-management
Vision therapy
Geriatrics
Environmental vision
Sports vision
Neuro-optometric rehabilitation
Nursing home eye care
Computers and vision

4 Accelerated orthokeratology

Robert C. Bauman, O.D., explains why accelerated orthokeratology is front and center in his Woodbury, CT, practice: "Not only has it been a great option for non-surgical vision correction for my patients, but this procedure has also given me a unique way to differentiate my practice from those of others. Fees are very lucrative and managed care, cost-containment constraints aren't an issue."[5]

5 Low vision services

"The number of individuals with vision loss from AMD and other disorders will double in the next 10 years," says Louis L. Lipschultz, O.D., Lithia Springs, GA. "Incorporating basic low vision services in a primary care practice can enhance the lives of many patients, increase revenue, differentiate your practice and provide an essential service."[6]

6 Therapeutic services

"A therapeutic practice takes years to develop," says John "Bucky" Gazaway, O.D., Eagle Grove, IA, "but it's worth every minute of time invested. I've grown my practice at a healthy rate in recent years—to the point where 60% of my revenue comes from treating disease and managing chronic conditions." He adds, "I don't have to schedule extra time for therapeutic visits, which usually take one-third to two-thirds less time than comprehensive exams. Yet, I earn up to twice as much for therapeutic visits than I do for traditional visits, and my patients are satisfied."[7]

7 Vision therapy

"By offering vision therapy as part of your primary care practice," says Daniel G. Bintz, O.D., Elk City, OK, "you will be opening a whole new world for your patients by giving them a service that can change their lives. Your patients will be loyal to you because you helped them in a way that no one else had been able to, and these services will open doors to new referrals. Starting with the basics and keeping overhead low, your net will increase without a large outlay of capital. In addition to the exam income, the satisfaction that comes with helping children and adults fulfill their potential in school and work is priceless."[8]

8 Computer vision syndrome testing

"By incorporating the CVS testing into our comprehensive exam," says Phil Smith, O.D., San Diego, CA, "we are uncovering a large number of patients whose symptoms can be easily minimized or eliminated with a pair of computer-specific eyeglasses. Providing superior computer vision care has resulted in some of our most satisfied patients and our greatest number of referrals."[9]

9 State-of-the-art equipment

"Patients are seeing and using technology in every aspect of their lives," says Gary Gerber, O.D., Hawthorne, NJ. "They have come to expect it at their eye doctor's office. So yes, it's not only worth it—it's now become a necessity." [10]

The benefits include improved diagnostic skills, greater productivity, higher fees, more referrals for tests that other O.D.s and M.D.s are unable to do, and a better image.

Neil B. Gailmard, O.D., M.B.A., F.A.A.O., Munster, IN, recommends developing a priority list of automated instruments that would benefit your practice. Then, invest in one each year, leasing or financing if necessary. Topping his list is an autoperimeter, followed by an autorefractor/keratometer, a retinal camera (preferably digital), a corneal topographer, a non-contact tonometer, and an AutoLensmeter.

Other "nice-to-have" instruments on his list include a nerve fiber analyzer and a scanning laser ophthalmoscope.

"One useful advantage of the scanning laser ophthalmoscope," says Dr. William L. Jones, O.D., Albuquerque, NM, "is that it's quick and patient friendly. You can have your technician capture a patient's image and send it almost immediately to the monitor in the exam room. By the time the patient comes in and sits down, you can have the image of the fundus up and on the screen." [11]

Another consideration: To the extent a scanning laser ophthalmoscope eliminates the need for dilation, it significantly reduces chair time. "Typically, dilating a patient is a five-step process that takes 1 hour and 40 minutes from the time the patient enters your office until he walks out," says Philip M. Buscemi, O.D. "This instrument requires a two-step process that takes 25 minutes, and the patient leaves driving." [12]

"If you're going to treat disease, you must invest in technology," says Eric E. Schmidt, O.D., Elizabethtown, NC. "For example, to treat glaucoma thoroughly, you need a visual field unit, a retinal thickness analyzer or nerve fiber analyzer, and a fundus camera. With these instruments, you can diagnose 99% of all glaucoma cases. Not only will this equipment set your practice apart, but it also will become a revenue center." [13]

"Pachymeters have four main applications for measuring corneal thickness," says Loretta Szczotka, O.D., M.S., F.A.A.O., director of the contact lens service at University Hospitals of Cleveland. "One would be LASIK; the second would be for contact lens swelling predominantly from extended wear; the third would be corneal thinning disorders, particularly keratoconus; and the fourth would be corneal swelling disorders, such as pseudophakic bullous keratopathy or Fuchs' dystrophy. Those are the four areas for which we use it most frequently." [14]

"To stay ahead of the game," says Marc R. Bloomenstein, O.D., F.A.A.O., Phoenix, AZ, "practitioners need to have all of the data in front of them before they make any recommendations to the patient. Pachymetry is a crucial step before LASIK, because if the cornea isn't thick enough, then you won't be able to perform the procedure comfortably. In this situation, other procedures may be recommended; for example, PRK, or an intraocular or phakic lens instead."[14]

10 Hard-learned lessons about equipment

- "When you upgrade your equipment," says Gregg L. Ossip, O.D., Indianapolis, IN, "you're also pushing the skills envelope of your staff. Not only have you increased your ability to delegate to a higher level of sophistication, you've added a new dimension of empowerment to your staffers. They're now providing the testing and care that previously only you could have provided."[15]
- "Embracing high-technology instrumentation," says Craig Andrews, O.D., Salem, IL, "has helped us grow to perhaps the largest optometric practice in southern Illinois, despite our being located in a small town in a largely rural area."[16]
- "In evaluating instruments," says Joseph T. Barr, O.D., M.S., F.A.A.O., Editor of *Contact Lens Spectrum*, "keep these factors in mind: How will it help my patients? How will it help my practice? How can I efficiently integrate its utility into my office? How fast can I pay for it? Can I test drive it in my office and not just at a meeting exhibit?"[17]

11 Laser surgery suite

It's a trend that most certainly differentiates an optometric practice: leasing or buying an excimer laser and bringing in a surgeon and specialized team to provide the whole service on-site in your practice.

FROM THE SUCCESS FILES

"When an O.D. brings a laser in-house," says R. Whitman Lord, O.D., Statesboro, GA, "his office, rather than the surgeon, gets credit for restoring the patient's vision. I've never witnessed more enthusiastic patients than next-day follow-up LASIK patients. Many patients tell us on their first follow-up visit that they'll be referring others."[18]

REALITY CHECK

Neil B. Gailmard, O.D., M.B.A., F.A.A.O., Munster, IN, says he does not "want a surgeon from a practice within easy driving distance due to the risk of losing referrals to that office. The surgeon he chose is based 2 hours away, which does not pull patients from his market area, yet is close enough in the event of complications."[18]

12 Meticulous about infection control measures

The risk for contamination in an optometric office is low, but discerning patients are nonetheless concerned about in-office prophylaxis. Some watch your every move.

"Does a staff member wipe surfaces with a disinfectant?" asks Peter G. Shaw-McMinn, O.D., F.A.A.O., Riverside, CA. "When you enter the exam room, do you first wash your hands in view of the patient to reinforce infection control?"[19]

13 Knowledgeable staff

The more knowledgeable and better trained your staff is, the more valuable they are to your practice and the more they help to differentiate it from rank-and-file offices.

Does your staff know, for example, what to say to patients who telephone with concerns about flashers and floaters, sudden vision loss, chemical splashes in the eye, foreign bodies, subconjunctival hemorrhage, or other injuries to the eyes?

Can your staff answer such common questions as follows: Why do you dilate my eyes? Can I have a copy of my prescription? What does this instrument do? If I'm seeing fine, why do I need to come in? Why can't I just order my lenses from a mail order company?

How well your staff fields questions about refractive surgery may be a deciding factor in whether a patient trusts you to help make this decision.

FROM THE SUCCESS FILES

"Hire a coordinator whose responsibilities are contact lenses and refractive surgery counseling," advises Paul M. Karpecki, O.D., Overland Park, KS. "It may cost more initially, but most doctors in a focus group of young doctors (who tripled practice growth over 10 years) said they've done this."

"When a patient says, 'I'm interested in refractive surgery,' you can say, 'I'll have my counselor talk to you about it.'"

If you co-manage one extra refractive surgery patient per week, says Dr. Karpecki, you will earn enough to pay the coordinator's salary three times over.[20]

David Shipley, O.D., maintains a low vision practice in Deerfield Beach, FL. "In addition to hiring trained employees who are well versed in low vision, he works with his staff regularly to update their knowledge. He employs an occupational therapist who works with physically impaired patients. If the patient has trouble holding a book, the occupational therapist can work with Dr. Shipley to devise a program that develops the patient's neuromuscular skills to complement the low vision acclimation."[21]

14 An office free of "architectural barriers"

The Americans with Disabilities Act requires businesses to be accessible to the disabled. Yet, many optometric offices have distant parking, stairs, and protruding thresholds or narrow entranceways that place restrictions on the accessibility of their offices for the 43 million Americans—more than one out of seven—who are physically disabled.

Compliance with Americans with Disabilities Act guidelines makes your practice more accessible to individuals with wheelchairs or other supportive devices, and the numbers are only increasing as more people are living longer and, in many cases, becoming mobility impaired.

Optometrists and staff members who understand and accommodate the needs of this sizable group will earn their goodwill and referrals as well as that of their families and friends.

15 Address the needs of deaf and hard-of-hearing patients

There are between 22 and 24 million Americans who are deaf or hard-of-hearing. Some have relatively minor difficulty hearing. Others are profoundly deaf and communicate with sign language, lip reading, written messages, or a combination of these methods.

FROM THE SUCCESS FILES

Beverly B. Miller, O.D., has built a specialty practice in the Washington, DC, area by addressing the needs of deaf and hard-of-hearing patients.

This area has a greater density of such patients than do many other parts of the country, partly because of nearby Gallaudet University for the deaf and hard-of-hearing and partly because of the great number of federal government employees who are deaf or hard-of-hearing.

The first step, says Dr. Miller, is to become fluent in sign language. "Luckily," she adds, "I was motivated because I have some deaf acquaintances."

Step two is to make your practice accessible to deaf and hard-of-hearing patients: They have to be able to call in and make their own appointments, and your staff has to be comfortable with that. This means installing a telecommunications device for the deaf (TDD) in your office, so patients can call and then type in their messages. In addition, Dr. Miller has offered courses in signing to her staff.

Step three is to get the word out. In the beginning, Dr. Miller spent most of her evenings, for approximately 1 year, giving lectures on general vision care to student groups at nearby Gallaudet University, as well as groups at Gallaudet's high school and elementary programs. She also alerted local school nurses to the special services she could provide to deaf and hard-of-hearing patients.

16 Curb appeal

In real estate jargon, *curb appeal* refers to the total impression a building creates from the street, including its overall condition, landscaping, and individual features. Curb appeal affects the market value of a building, its salability, as well as the *image* of its occupants—for better or for worse.

Among the elements that produce a negative curb appeal are any of the following:

- A parking lot with cracked pavement, overgrown weeds, or discarded items
- An outdoor sign in need of repair, repainting, or replacement
- Poor outdoor lighting (especially important for a practice with evening hours)
- Exterior paint that is peeling, blistered, stained, or faded
- Masonry that needs to be repointed
- Trees or shrubs in need of pruning, spraying, or replacement
- Windows with cracked or dirty panes
- A roof with missing shingles
- Wilted plants or flowers
- An unsightly doorway

ACTION STEPS

It's all too easy to grow accustomed to small flaws that diminish a building's curb appeal. Seek a fresh perspective by asking your staff, or perhaps several of your best patients, to evaluate the building's exterior as if they were seeing it for the first time. Are there overlooked problems? Is the curb appeal in tune with your target population? What recommendations would they have to improve the building's curb appeal?

Such feedback may prove useful in the negotiations to renew your lease, and perhaps in deciding whether to relocate. If you own the building, it may motivate you to make the needed improvements.

17   An appealing, up-to-date office

What kind of image does your office convey, and is it congruent with the level of professionalism you want to project and the quality of care you provide? The fact is, you don't have a choice as to whether your office makes a statement or not; your only choice is what kind of statement.

HARD-LEARNED LESSON

Every seven years, you need to either redecorate or move. If you don't notice the sameness, your patients will.

In a survey of its National Panel, *Review of Optometry* found that among 244 respondents, the average doctor has been in the same office 14 years. Four in 10 say they will renovate something this year. Sixty-seven percent expect to spend $10,000–$25,000; 12%, $25,000–$50,000; and the remaining doctors of optometry varying amounts of $50,000 or more.

If money were no object, the changes on these respondents' "wish lists" were as follows[22]:

Change furnishings and décor (54%)
Add exam lanes (47%)
Expand dispensary (34%)
Reconfigure floor plan (39%)
Upgrade reception area (38%)
Upgrade or add employee amenities (25%)
Add parking (17%)
Add an in-office lab (16%)
Get a personal office (15%)
Move (15%)

HARD-LEARNED LESSON FOR THE NEW DOCTOR OF OPTOMETRY

I saw a sign in an interior decorator's office in Portland, OR, that read "The longer your office says struggling attorney, the longer the struggle."

18 Don't overlook this room

There is one room in particular that gets noticed and evaluated more often than you might guess and not just by patients, but by *staff* as well—the *bathroom*.

The complaints include old fixtures, a small mirror, poor lighting, and (most seriously) "dirty."

Take a new look at your office bathroom. What, if anything, does it communicate about your practice? The importance you place on quality, cleanliness, and attention to detail? What message does it send your *staff*?

Keeping the bathroom *spotlessly clean* is a must, regardless of cost.

If indicated, consider remodeling the bathroom from top to bottom with new, color-coordinated fixtures; a large, well-lighted mirror; attractive wallpaper; and designer perfumes. Go the whole way. Your patients will like it and your staff will *love* it, guaranteed.

Ask your staff for ideas. Better yet, if they have the interest, give them a budget and let them plan everything.

If the job entails remodeling, consider providing at least one large stall with railings for wheelchair patients. Levers instead of round handles on doors and water faucets are also helpful to arthritic patients.

FROM THE SUCCESS FILES

Cynthia F. Kleppinger M.D., family physician in Hagerstown, MD, believes patients like a homey, personal touch in the office. "I placed a shadow box on the wall of our lavatory facility," she writes, "and pictures of children playing. A basket of dried flowers is near the sink, and I have a pretty cover for the tissue box. My patients appreciate the extra touches, and I like the way the lavatory looks, too."[23]

19 A friendly staff

One of the first things patients notice about a practice is the *ambiance*. An upbeat, friendly staff is a huge plus for a practice, especially in today's "sign in–sit down–shut up" healthcare environment. And it is never an accident.

Friendliness is usually easy to spot. One of the signs is the number of times a job candidate *smiles* during the interview.

Nordstrom, the retailer based in Seattle, is famous for its friendly employees, but no special program made them that way. "When companies ask us if we'd like to come out and talk about our program, we just don't have a lot to say," a spokeswoman, Brooke White, said. "There's no great science to this. Mostly, we just think we're making good hiring decisions."[24]

20 Language fluency

Current statistics indicate that 11% of the U.S. population speaks a language at home other than English, and the number is increasing.

If, like many communities in the country, yours has significant numbers of non– or limited–English-speaking people with whom neither you nor your staff are able to converse, your practice is at a terrible disadvantage, especially if other practices have multilingual personnel.

ACTION STEPS

- Hire associates and/or staff members fluent in the language of the target populations you would like to attract to your office.
- If you are near a college or university, hire an exchange student for part-time work in your office as an interpreter.
- Offer to pay the tuition for a staff member willing to take an adult education course in the language needed for your practice—125% of the costs for an "A" in the course—and, on completion of it, give the person a raise.

- The book *Practical Spanish in Eye Care* (Butterworth–Heinemann, 2001) written by Brian Chou O.D., F.A.A.O., can get you started. It has 25 chapters covering general communication, history taking, all aspects of an examination, explanations of specific conditions, a Spanish-English vocabulary, and a guide to pronunciation.
- Another do-it-yourself resource: Audio-Forum offers 285 audio-cassette courses in 103 different languages. These vary in length from one and one-half hours (key phrases and vocabulary only) to 15–20 hours of recorded material. (A catalog of self-instructional language courses is available from: Audio-Forum, 96 Broad Street, Guilford, CT 06437; (800) 243-1234. Web site: http://www. audioforum.com)

FROM THE SUCCESS FILES

- Marc M. Berson, O.D., M.B.A., writes, "In our office in downtown Allentown, PA, we have a high percentage of Spanish-speaking patients. To accommodate this population, we have employed a fantastic, personable Spanish-speaking optician for more than 10 years. The loyalty these patients have to our practice is priceless."[25]
- "Ten years ago, I began practicing in Newport News, VA," says internist Brooks A. Mick, M.D., "amid the largest concentration of military posts in the world. Because of service personnel who married overseas and former military people who've tended to settle in this area, there are many folks here whose primary language is Korean, Vietnamese, Japanese, Spanish, or Tagalog (Filipino). I try to greet each patient in his or her own language, and it has become something of a ritual to ask every patient who speaks a new language to teach me a few words. It's remarkable how much goodwill a single phrase can promote."[26]
- At the Children's Dental Building in Artesia, CA, the following sign is posted:

We Speak Your Language

"Our staff is experienced with Spanish, Portuguese, Tagalog, Japanese, Chinese, Vietnamese, Farsi, and Sign Language. We're here to help."

The facility also has a TDD phone for the hearing impaired.

21   Extended hours

Because of job pressures and time constraints, fewer people than ever are able (or want) to take time off from work for an eye examination. Extended office hours, whether in the morning or evening, possibly both, have become if not an imperative, at least an important consideration, especially if other offices have them.

REALITY CHECK

"Many managed care plans require their panel members to work evenings and weekends," says Allen D. Leck, former President of Primary Eyecare Network in San Ramon, CA. In addition, "Owing to the increased activity and locations of the chains, it is becoming essential for practitioners to keep their offices open additional hours just to compete."[27]

Note: If you have evening hours, make sure the parking lot at your building is well lit.

If you're not sure whether your patients would prefer extended hours in the morning or the evening, ask them (see Chapter 8).

Early morning hours attract what many optometrists refer to as "no nonsense" patients, often more concerned with time than money. So, they're in and out and on their way. Many practitioners report these early-hour appointments are among the most popular and productive of the day—and are booked far in advance.

FROM THE SUCCESS FILES

"On Thursdays, I start my workday at 6:30 a.m. and end it at 2:00 p.m.," says Albert L. Ousborne, Jr., D.D.S., Towson, MD. "This allows our 'early-riser patients' an opportunity to come in prior to work. We've had only one opening in the five years since we started at this hour."[28]

Before-school appointments for children also tend to be more productive than after-school appointments. The reason: Children are more rested and better behaved.

In a poll by the Gallup Organization, 77% of the women and 67% of the men interviewed said they are more productive in the mornings than in the afternoons.

How about you? If you're a morning person, give some thought to starting earlier. You'll accommodate those patients who prefer early morning appointments, and because it is your "best" time of day, you'll also greatly increase your productivity.

22 Transportation to the office

In every community, there are people for whom getting to a doctor's office is difficult, if not impossible. Some no longer drive or have an automobile or don't wish to impose on neighbors to drive them, wait, and then drive them home again. They don't live near public transportation, and if they do, they're often reluctant to use it. The number of people in these situations is increasing because of an aging population.

Your office can help such patients (including those scheduled for in-office refractive surgery or even a dilated exam) by considering the following:

A courtesy vehicle (owned by the practice) can be used to pick up and return home those patients unable to get to the office in any other way. Included are teenagers with appointments after school and with no means of transportation (other than a bicycle). Parents will be most appreciative.

Another option: taxi rides for such patients (at your expense).

Call your local Office on Aging or Senior Center facility to learn about free or low-cost transportation services (e.g., van, taxi, or volunteer drivers), which many communities offer.

FROM THE SUCCESS FILES

At the office of Nancy Andree, D.D.S., Waco, TX, an office sign reads, "Anyone having trouble getting transportation to our office? Give us a call and we'll send our *Toothmobile* to get you."

TESTED TIP

Check with your insurance carrier to make sure you have the proper coverage for such a service.

23 On time for appointments

Being "on time" gives your practice a competitive advantage in today's time-pressured environment. It sends a message as well because in our society, time spent waiting is linked to *status*. The more important you are, the more promptly you're seen. VIPs never wait.

Martha Zarnow, a vice president of Viacom International, was quoted in the *Wall Street Journal* on why she fired her obstetrician after an extended stay in his waiting room: "I'm a busy professional," she said. "I don't make people wait for me and I don't expect to be kept waiting. Whenever I notice that kind of arrogance, I switch doctors."[29]

REALITY CHECK

How long will patients remain good-natured about waiting beyond their appointment time? The answer: 15 minutes, according to a study of 10,000 patients interviewed by National Research Corporation of Lincoln, NE.

HARD-LEARNED LESSONS ABOUT WAITING

- Anxiety makes waiting seem longer.
- Uncertain waits are longer than known, finite waits.
- Unexplained waits are longer than explained waits.
- Unfair waits are longer than equitable waits.
- When you do fall behind schedule, a sincere "I'm sorry you had to wait so long" really does have a mellowing effect.

24 Mobile optometry clinic

A few years ago, Roger Pabst, O.D., chair of the American Optometric Association's VISION USA program, and his partners in Southwest Minnesota's PBR Optometric Clinic considered how many elderly people in nearby towns were without immediate access to eye and vision care. As a result, they came up with a common-sense solution to the problem: "Rather than transporting patients to eye care, bring eye care to the patients," observed Dr. Pabst. Soon after, the PBR Optometric Mobile Eye Clinic was created.

Since 1995, Dr. Pabst and the PBR Optometric Mobile Eye Clinic have offered state-of-the-art eye and vision care to nursing facility residents and other older adults in 11 small Minnesota communities. The 37-foot, fully equipped mobile eye clinic operates on a limited schedule between May and September, serving facilities within a 60- to 70-mile radius of PBR's more conventional practices in the towns of Mt. Lake, Redwood Falls, Springfield, Tracy, and Windom.

"It's not a money maker as such," Dr. Pabst says. "We get the standard Medicaid (or in some cases, Medicare) reimbursement. However, we do not charge extra to bring the mobile unit. That's an added expense on our part. But the rewards of serving the older adult population with a mobile optometry clinic are not all monetary. I just feel that there's a need out there."[30]

25 Child-friendly

"When your office is the one that provides vision care for children, you set yourself apart," says Elliot J. Klonsky, O.D., Crofton, MO.

"Parents truly appreciate doctors," he adds, "who make their children (and themselves) feel comfortable. In many cases, the parents are more anxious than the children about how the office visit will go."[31]

"What may be routine to you," adds David G. Kirschen, O.D., Ph.D., Brea, CA, "may be very frightening to the child. Try to put him or her at ease, even if you must talk funny, act like a clown, or use humor and exaggeration."[32]

FROM THE SUCCESS FILES

The following form used by the Department of Dentistry at the Illinois Masonic Medical Center in Chicago is sent to parents in advance of a child's first visit. The brief introduction explains its one and only purpose.

Pre-Need Questionnaire for Children

The purpose of this questionnaire is to learn more about your child before beginning his/her dental care. Your answers will help to make your child's visits to the dentist more predictable and productive.

1. Is this your child's first visit to a dental office?   Yes   No
2. If not, how would you describe your child's previous visits?
3. How long is your child's attention span at home (other than TV watching)?
4. Does your child have any pets, hobbies, special interests, or recent accomplishments? If yes, please list:
5. Is there any additional information that might help us in treating your child?

QUESTIONS TO CONSIDER

- Would the information from such a questionnaire (modified for optometry) help, as the form says, to make a child's first visit "more predictable and productive"?
- What impression do you think this pre-need questionnaire would make on the parent(s) receiving it before the child's first visit?
- Does it convey a "child-friendly" image?

ADDITIONAL TIP

The Wyoming Optometric Association's Web site (http://www.wyoming. optometry.net) has a page about "Children's Vision." It includes several tips for parents to make their child's optometric examination a positive experience: "(1) Make an appointment early in the day. Allow about one hour. (2) Talk about the examination in advance and encourage your child's questions. (3) Explain the examination in your child's terms, comparing the E chart to a puzzle and the instruments to tiny flashlights and a kaleidoscope."

---

26 Answer patients' questions

One of the most frequent complaints that today's patients have about visits to their doctors is *the feeling of being rushed.* Is it because of managed care? Is it the need for greater productivity? Is it a faulty perception?

REALITY CHECK

A study by the University of California—Irvine Medical School showed that physicians don't spend as much time with patients as they think they do. Doctors believe they spend an average of 12 minutes giving information to patients while the *actual time* spent averages *only 1.3 minutes.*

FROM THE SUCCESS FILES

I recently interviewed a physician who had posted the following letters on the back of his exam room door:

I.T.A.E.Y.W.L.T.A.M.

"The letters," he said, "are a reminder to ask every patient before leaving the room, *Is there anything else you would like to ask me?*"

"Does that open the door," I asked, "for a lot of questions that might be time consuming to answer?"

"Surprisingly, not very often," he replied. "Most times, it's a question the patient intended to ask but forgot, and it's easily answered. When it's a question that requires a lengthy answer, I either give the patient some literature that has the necessary information, ask a qualified staff person to answer the question, or perhaps set up another appointment to discuss the matter in more depth."

Asking patients if they have any questions at the conclusion of an office visit sends positive messages that will be appreciated. It will also help differentiate your practice from high-volume, assembly-line practitioners who are often too busy and too time pressured to answer patients' questions.

TIP

Asking I.T.A.E.Y.W.L.T.A.M. while standing in the doorway of the exam room with your hand on the doorknob conveys a strong message that you don't really want questions. They're the right words, but that's the wrong body language.

ANOTHER OPTION

Let new patients know *before* they ever get to your office that you're willing to answer questions and that your practice is indeed different from the one(s) they may have previously left.

Consider having your receptionist say to patients calling for a first appointment: "If you have any questions to ask the doctor, write them down and bring the list with you. We'll make sure all of your questions are answered." The gesture alone will be appreciated.

27 Listen, really listen, to patients

Related to spending adequate time with patients and answering questions is the importance of listening to patients in a skillful and understanding way. "It reduces your risk of exposure to malpractice claims," says New York City attorney Andrew Feldman, who often defends healthcare providers in such matters. Among his recommendations are the following:

- Pay attention when a patient speaks.
- *Look* like you're paying attention. Looking, for example, at a patient's chart, or worse, your watch, implies less-than-total interest on your part. Someone worth listening *to* is worth looking *at*.
- Get involved while listening. Don't be a deadpan. Lean forward. Nod your head as the patient speaks. Respond to the patient's cues and facial expressions. Periodically say "uh-huh," "that's interesting," or other words to show you're listening.
- Paraphrase or summarize what you've understood the patient to have said—it lets patients know you've correctly heard the message. And, if you haven't, it enables you and the patient to achieve clarity. Such responses are time consuming but help ensure that two-way communication takes place.
- Finally, before concluding the patient's visit, always ask: "Is there anything else you would like to ask me?"

"This dialoging back and forth," Mr. Feldman says, "is important, not only for its clinical significance, but also as a secondary benefit, a means to minimize your exposure to malpractice claims."

28 Thoroughness

Many optometrists take justifiable pride in the thoroughness of their comprehensive examinations and report how often patients say, "that's the most thorough exam I've ever had."

Siret Jaanus, Ph.D., F.A.A.O., a professor of pharmacology at the State University of New York College of Optometry and co-editor of *Clinical Ocular Pharmacology* (Butterworth–Heinemann, 2001) advises eye care professionals to delve deeper into patients' medical and medication histories: "You should find out exactly what diseases your patients are being treated for, and get a complete drug history that includes all prescriptions and over-the-counter medications they are taking and have previously taken—including the dosage of each drug and how long it's been taken." If your history or examination reveals possible drug side effects, you have an obligation to step in. "Either in writing or verbally, you should consult with the treating physician. A lower drug dose or, if possible, prescribing a different drug may help to prevent serious visual problems."[33]

REALITY CHECK

Thoroughness is commendable and an important way to differentiate your practice. Beware, however, of spending more time than necessary.

Neil B. Gailmard, O.D., M.B.A., F.A.A.O., Munster, IN, says, "Realize that patients don't want an eye exam to take a long time. Doctors equate length with quality. Patients don't."[34]

29 Available for emergencies

FROM THE SUCCESS FILES

Robert L. Simmons, O.D., Clinton, IA, like many high-performance optometrists, is available 24 hours a day, 7 days a week—not only for his patients, but also for the emergency room at the local hospital. The goodwill from both patients and physicians, he says, has been incalculable and has resulted in many referrals.

Consider also notifying hotels, pharmacies, and school nurses of your availability in the event of an emergency.

30 Participate in clinical research

Long involved with solution and contact lens studies, Bobby Christensen, O.D., F.A.A.O., Midwest City, OK, cites numerous benefits of clinical studies.

- "Sharpens my clinical skills by requiring me to observe subtle changes, such as protein accumulation on lens surfaces, epithelial damage, and topography changes owing to mechanical pressure and hypoxia."
- "Clinical trials help us standardize office records for grading injection, staining, edema, protein buildup, giant papillary conjuctivitis, etc."

"The patients who are selected to participate in these studies," says Dr. Christensen, "are loyal to the practice and are some of our best referral sources. I believe," he adds, "that many patients seek doctors who they perceive as cutting-edge providers."[35]

31 Be senior-friendly

According the National Center for Health Statistics, nearly 37% of all visits to doctors' offices for eye care are made by persons 65 years of age and older who now represent 13% of the U.S. population. In the year 2011, 76 million Baby Boomers will begin turning 65. The "Age Wave" is upon us.

"As the population ages, it's important for optometrists working with elderly patients to be aware of the issues associated with vision loss as part of the aging process," says Alfred A. Rosenbloom Jr., M.A., O.D., D.O.S., chair emeritus of the Low Vision Service of the Chicago Lighthouse and former president of the Illinois College of Optometry. "Older people have various reactions to the onset of vision loss, as well as the recognition of further vision loss over time. These may range from denial that vision loss has occurred to acceptance and readiness to learn adaptive techniques for carrying out various tasks of daily living. The support of professionals and significant others is essential so that steps toward rehabilitation services can be made."[36]

At the Hunterdon Medical Center in Flemington, NJ, medical residents spend 3 hours learning how it feels to be old. "A makeup artist deepens the lines on their face, adds gray to their hair, and powders a pallor onto their skin. They are given yellowed contact lenses with a smearing of Vaseline to blur their vision, they don rubber gloves to dim their sense of touch, and they wear wax earplugs to diminish their hearing. Splints are fastened to their joints, making it difficult to move. Raw peas in their shoes simulate corns and calluses.

"With their limitations in place, they are sent to several departments in the hospital. In the x-ray clinic, the residents are sent into small changing rooms and told to undress, then redress. At the pharmacy, they are required to fill out Medicaid insurance forms in order to receive a variety of prescriptions. They then return to the program training room, where they are assigned a variety of seemingly simple tasks: thread a needle, read the label and open the child-proof caps on the medicine vials, open an orange juice container, unwrap the plastic from a bran muffin.

"In addition to increasing the sensitivity of those who work with the elderly," says Linda F. Bryant, coordinator of the program, "this training has brought visible changes to the hospital. Signs have been made easier to read, registration counters have been lowered to wheelchair height, and elevator doors have been altered to allow slower-moving patients more time to get on and off."[37]

As practitioners of the healing arts, let's listen, smile, extend a helping hand, and give the respect due to older patients. Remember, we're next in line.

32 E.T.D.B.W.

Consultant Michael Hammer in his book, *The Agenda: What Every Business Must Do to Dominate the Decade* (Crown Business, 2001), writes that companies must do better jobs of organizing themselves around the process of satisfying customers. First and foremost, he says, they have to be E.T.D.B.W. (*easy to do business with*).

"We want to make it easier and easier for our customers to do business with us," says Bill Price, vice president of global customer service for Amazon.com. "We want to have everything go so right, you never have to contact us. To do that, we have to stay tuned up. We have to keep asking, What are the problems?"[38]

How can optometrists be easy to do business with?

- If patients call because of an "emergency" or what they *perceive* as an emergency, have the receptionist simply ask, "How soon can you get here?"
- The following sign from the staff lounge of a busy orthopedic practice indicates the enlightened approach many physicians have taken toward emergency patients: "When a person calls requesting an appointment for the same day of the call, do not turn him or her away without first running it by Camille or Harriet (office manager and treatment coordinator) or one of the doctors. Depending on the symptoms, they will either talk with the patient or make the determination as to whether or not he or she should be seen."
- If a patient calls to change an appointment, even if it's at the last minute, have the receptionist *just do it*. A long sigh or sign of annoyance will accomplish nothing. Patients who have repeated difficulties in keeping appointments in the office of Marvin Mansky, D.D.S., New York, NY, are requested to call on the day they'd like to come in. "If we have the time," he says, "we're glad to see them."
- If a patient requests a copy of their eyeglass prescription, give it to them (Federal Trade Commission Ruling 456.2 requires it).
- Have your staff help patients in any way they can with the determination of their insurance benefits and the filing of the necessary forms. A sign in the staff lounge of one office reads: "Please do not be

abusive to patients with insurance problems. They're 75% of our practice."

- Do anything to please a patient. Anthony Leach, O.D., Chattanooga, TN, offers a dramatic example. "A patient who had spent $600 on eyewear stopped in the office." Dr. Leach asked how she liked her glasses. She said she wasn't sure she made the best choice. He promptly remade the glasses in another expensive frame, at no charge. "It cost us something," he says, "but it brought us more. That patient is really happy now, and she'll never leave us."[39]
- How about refunds? "In the final analysis," says consultant Jerry Hayes, O.D., "I think it's a mistake in this competitive environment to have a hard and fast policy that you don't give refunds. For exams, I'd consider refunds in the rare case that someone is just plain not satisfied. For the unhappy purchaser of glasses or contact lenses, I'd recommend that you make a policy of giving credits, if not refunds."[40]

FROM THE SUCCESS FILES

"Our premise is simple," says Elizabeth Spaulding, vice president of customer satisfaction, L. L. Bean Inc. "If a product doesn't meet a customer's expectations, whatever they may be, we will replace it, repair it, or refund the customer's money. The point is, the customer determines the expectation. Not us."[41]

ACTION STEP

Schedule a staff meeting to discuss various ways to make your practice E.T.D.B.W. It will heighten everyone's awareness of this important strategy to differentiate your practice and give it a substantial and sustainable competitive edge.

33 Be consistent

- Does out-of-date equipment imply out-of-date knowledge and skills?
- Does an office that is anything less than meticulously clean cast suspicions on the quality of care?

- Can a receptionist who gives patients a hard time about seeing the doctor in an "emergency" or changing appointments "sour" them against your practice?

Perhaps not. But to many people, these inconsistencies send negative messages. The reason? People tend to judge the unknown by the known. It emphasizes the need for consistency between the image you *want* your practice to project to others and the image it *does* project.

If you want to communicate a message of "quality care," then everything in your practice and everything you, your associates, and your staff members do must exude *quality*—clearly, compellingly, and *consistently*.

FROM THE SUCCESS FILES

"Our practice isn't the least expensive or the most convenient in our area," says S. Barry Eiden, O.D., F.A.A.O., Chicago, IL, "yet we're in the top 5–10% of American optometric practices in revenue generated. We show sustained growth in all aspects of practice at a time when the productivity of many private practices and corporate vision centers is stagnating or declining. I believe we owe our success to our patients' belief that our quality of care, expertise, experience and value exceed our competition's."[42]

34 SuperService

"Consider the enormous challenge facing any company attempting to differentiate itself in the marketplace," says George Gendron, Editor of *Inc.* "With reduced barriers to entry and a flood of new competitors, virtually all of our core products and services have been turned into commodities. Providing state-of-the-art customer service is one of the few means left for a company to help itself stand out from the crowd."[43]

This editorial was not aimed at optometrists, but the prescription for differentiating your practice in a commoditized marketplace is the same: ensuring that patients experience a uniformly high level of service throughout their interactions with your practice. In a word, it is providing what I call *SuperService.*

What is *SuperService*? It can be summed up in three words: *and then some*. It means doing what patients expect you to do—and then some.

---

35 Secret of the Philadelphia hoagie

Reminiscing about his early life in Philadelphia, Joel Novack, D.P.M. (now practicing in Cleveland, OH), recalled the sensational hoagies (hero) sandwiches made by a local chain of delicatessens. On one occasion, he asked the proprietor what made their hoagies so much better than those made by other delis.

"Is it the crusty bread?" Dr. Novack asked.

"No," the proprietor replied.

"Is it the special meats and cheeses?"

Again, the answer was "no."

"How about the olive oil? The condiments?"

"No," the proprietor said, "It's *everything*."

"That simple lesson," Dr. Novack says, "made a lasting impression. And, years later, I realized the same principle applies to practice. It's no one thing that leads to success. It's *everything*—starting from the moment the patient first calls the office. It's how they're spoken to by staff members and doctors, how their concerns are addressed, or how their insurance coverage is handled. It's whether patients see signs of competence and caring during their office visit or an assembly-line attitude. It's whether they see a neat, spotlessly clean, well-equipped office or something less."

True differentiation in an endeavor seldom results from doing just one thing that much better than anyone else: *It comes from doing 100 things just 1% better.*

Notes

1. Tenuta CD. What Makes Your Practice Special? *Rehab Economics*, March 2001, 42.
2. Healthy Patients, Healthy Practices. Supplement to *Optometric Management*, July 2001, 7S.

3. Eisenberg JS. LASIK in 2010: Will You Be There? *Review of Optometry,* October 15, 2000, 54–62.

4. Winslow C. Put Your Practice in a League of Its Own. *Review of Optometry,* August 1993, 31–32,36.

5. Bauman RC. A Night and Day Difference, Part 1. *Optometric Management,* April 2001, 57–59,77.

6. Lipschultz LL. Making Your Practice Low-Vision Friendly. *Optometric Management,* July 2001, 114.

7. Gazaway J "Bucky." Debunking the Myths: How One O.D. Thrives with Therapeutics. *Optometric Management,* August 1998, 12S.

8. Bintz DG, Bither M. Practical Vision Therapy in a Primary Care Practice. *Practical Optometry,* April 1999, 64–78.

9. Smith P. Computer Vision Care: An Opportunity We Can't Afford to Miss. *California Optometry,* September/October 1998, 12–13.

10. Black A. It's an e-World Techno-Explosion. *Review of Optometry,* November 2000, 63–68.

11. Jones WL. A View of the Retina: Wider Is Better. *Review of Optometry,* June 2001, 79–82.

12. Buscemi PM. A Wider Field of View. *Optometric Management,* June 2001, 42,44.

13. Schmidt EE. Rx for Success. *Optometric Management,* August 2001, 12–13.

14. Watson D. Pachymetry Best Serves Contact Lens-Based, Surgical Co-Management Practices. *Primary Care Optometry News,* October 2001, 17–19.

15. Ossip GL. Getting Wired. *Optometric Management,* March 1997, 49,51,53–54.

16. Andrews C. High-Tech Diagnostic Instrumentation Improves Patient Care. *Optometry Today,* April 1995, 28–30.

17. Barr JT. Instrumentation for Your Practice. *Contact Lens Spectrum,* August 2001, 13.

18. Gailmard NB. Moving LASIK to the Forefront of Your Practice. *Optometric Management,* February 2001, 53–58.

19. Shaw-McMinn P. Achieving Patient Retention. *Optometric Management,* April 2001, 84–89.

20. Karpecki PM. Secrets to Successful Co-Management. *Optometric Management,* February 1999, 8S–10S.

21. Lamperelli K. Itch to Niche. *Review of Optometry,* March 15, 2001, 65–68,89.

22. Murphy J. How O.D.s Fix Their Offices. *Review of Optometry,* March 2000, 53–55.

23. Kleppinger CF. Add a Homey Touch. *Physician's Management,* February 1989, 25.

24. Murray K. Make Nice and Make It Snappy: Companies Try Courtesy Training, *New York Times*, April 2, 1995, Section 3.
25. Berson MM. Make Managed Care Work for You. *Primary Care Optometry News*, January 2001, 6.
26. Mick BA. Your Voices. *Medical Economics*, February 19, 2001, 96.
27. Leck AD. Point/Counterpoint. *Optometry Today*, July 1996, 12.
28. Ousborne AL Jr. Viewpoint. *Dental Economics*, August 2000, 12,14.
29. Zarnow M. OBG Management. *Monitor*, December 1994, 19.
30. Pabst R. Optometry on the Road. *Optometry*, May 2001, 333–334.
31. Klonsky E. Long-Term Practice Growth and the Pediatric Patient. *Optometry Today*, January/February 1994, 37.
32. Kirschen DG. The Special Patient: Get Started with Patients Just Getting Started in Life. *Review of Optometry*, January 2002, 48–55.
33. Payne K. Medications Commonly Associated with Ocular Side Effects. *http://www.sightstreet.com*, July 11, 2001.
34. Gailmard NB. Why Practices Don't Grow. *Optometric Management*, May 2000, 48,52,54.
35. Christensen B. Rx for Success. *Optometric Management*, October 2000, 95,97.
36. Rosenbloom AA Jr. Vision in the Elderly: More Than a Medical Issue. *Primary Care Optometry News*, March 2001, 24,26–27.
37. Belkin L. In Lessons on Empathy, Doctors Become Patients. *New York Times*, June 4, 1992, A1,B5.
38. Fishman C. But Wait, You Promised . . . *Fast Company*, April 2001, 110.
39. Lee J. How to Court Private Payers. *Review of Optometry*, April 2001, 29.
40. Hayes J. Do Refunds Make Sense? *Optometric Management*, March 2000, 24.
41. McCauley L. How May I Help You? *Fast Company*, March 2000, 93.
42. Eiden SB. The Proactive Therapeutic Approach. *Optometric Management*, September 2001, 92–97.
43. Gendron G. Standout Service. *Inc.*, April 2001, 11.

2

Long-Range, Strategic Planning

Strategic planning is the fundamental process by which an organization determines specific action steps to achieve future goals. It's the map to guide your activities on the way to your destination by identifying what needs to be done, by whom, with what resources, and by what date. Planning allows the organization as a whole to focus on the right priorities and activities to accomplish its goals and is one of the key management activities that allows an organization to proactively manage its growth.

Strategic planning starts with figuring out where you and your practice are headed; where you will be a year or two from now; and how you'll get there. Will the focus be the same? How about the priorities? Will you be serving the same patient base or entirely different segments of the population? Will you continue to offer the same mix of services and products or shift gears?

The answers to such questions influence everything in your practice, starting with *how* you do *what* you do, the kinds of patients you attract, your standards for quality and service, the location of your office, your fees, equipment, continuing education, whom you hire, the size of your staff, how you promote the practice, the pace of the practice, the overhead, and so on.

There is no "correct" answer as such. What's best for *you* depends on your needs, interests, priorities, and answers to the many questions posed in this book.

36 Conduct a S.W.O.T. analysis

A *S.W.O.T. analysis* is an important component of long-range, strategic planning that's widely used in industry. S.W.O.T. is an acronym for Strengths, Weaknesses, Opportunities, and Threats. A critical assessment of these issues is essential to develop an action plan for the future growth of your practice.

Strengths refer to the things you and your staff do exceptionally well, possibly better than anyone else. Or, perhaps there is something about your practice that gives it a competitive advantage, such as your location, high-tech equipment, unique services, office hours, caliber of personnel, contact lens inventory, or any of a host of other things. You need to know what these strengths are and make sure to maintain them.

FROM THE SUCCESS FILES

Eric E. Schmidt, O.D., Elizabethtown, NC, recalls, "As Director of a large optometric referral center in New Orleans, I'd already built a reputation in treating eye diseases. I wanted to continue treating ocular diseases, so when it came time to open my own practice, I knew choosing the right location could make or break the practice."

"I chose a retirement area in the southeastern part of the country," he says, "which is a hotbed for diseases such as diabetes and glaucoma. Then I tailored the practice to my objectives and stuck to the game plan."[1]

To help identify your strengths, discuss with your staff such questions as the following:

- What has made our practice successful?
- Why do patients bypass other practices, especially those with lower fees, to come to us?
- Are we best known for our medical, refractive, or optical services?
- Why do physicians and other professional people refer patients to our office?
- What accounts for patient loyalty?
- What are we most proud of?

One of the *strengths* that high-performance optometric practices invariably have in common is *outstanding service*, both clinically and optically.

REALITY CHECK

Most optometric practices have peaks and valleys: exceptionally busy times when there's not quite enough staff to always provide outstanding service, and slower times when there's more than enough staff to do a first-rate job.

Because it's next to impossible to be properly staffed at all times, which alternative then makes the most sense: To be (slightly) *understaffed* for the busy times, or (slightly) *overstaffed* for the slow times?

FROM THE SUCCESS FILES

- In the opinion of Neil Gailmard, O.D., M.B.A., F.A.A.O., Munster, IN, "The traditional benchmark of keeping staff compensation to 18% of the practice gross is outdated today. In fact," he adds, "I advise doctors to try to exceed 18%. This is the only way to provide outstanding service and to efficiently delegate office and clinical procedures. An excellent staff is one of the best investments you can make."[2]
- "To delegate successfully," says Walter S. Ramsey, O.D., F.A.A.O., Charleston, WV, "you must start with good people. I hire the very best employees I can find, although I have to pay far more than the average optometry practice does for personnel. If you always hire the best-qualified people, they'll pay for themselves in the long run."[3]
- Robert T. Moore, D.V.M., Wilson, NC, simply put it this way: "We're staffed for the *busiest* times—not the *slowest*."

The rationale behind this strategy is quality care + outstanding service (at all times) = greater patient satisfaction + loyalty + referrals = above-average practice growth.

Weaknesses refer to anything that has an adverse effect on productivity, profitability, patient satisfaction, and practice growth. These may include the following:

Things you're doing that you *shouldn't* be doing, such as long waits in the office, high-pressure tactics in the dispensary, overbooking and then rushing patients, and perhaps most importantly, cutting corners to improve profitability.

Things you need to do *more* of, such as continuing education, delegation, staff meetings, patient education, networking with physicians, and market research.

Aspects of your practice that you may have let *slip*, such as service, timely reports to physicians and other referral sources, office décor, staff training, addition of new equipment, collections, recalls, and the dispensary.

REALITY CHECK

Cost containment has its place, especially in today's managed-care environment of lowered reimbursements. When you start cutting corners, however, you have to be careful not to compromise such things as the quality of patient care, quality of materials, caliber of auxiliary personnel, level of service, equipment, office décor, continuing education, patient satisfaction, image, and, in the final analysis, practice growth.

The focus of this book is giving each of these factors the *highest priority* and *best efforts* of you and your staff—not cutting corners in any way. Hopefully, we're on the same page.

HARD-LEARNED LESSON

The key to success isn't cost containment—it's *revenue enhancement*.

Opportunities refer to what you could be doing (that you're not yet doing) or what you could be doing *differently* (than you're now doing) to achieve revenue enhancement and practice growth. This part of the analysis is so important and has so many possible options that an entire chapter has been devoted to it (Chapter 3).

Threats refer to any issue that may prevent you and your staff from reaching the goals you've set for your practice. To help identify these issues, consider such questions as the following:

- What is the "competition" doing in terms of services offered, equipment, hours of operation, professional fees, participation in third-party plans, and advertising?
- How does the eyewear selection, contact lens inventory, prices, guarantees, and delivery time in other offices compare with yours?

REALITY CHECK

Recently, I visited an optometrist in the southeast who told me about a relatively new practice approximately 2 miles away that was "clobbering" his well-regarded but aging practice and to which a sizable number of his patients had transferred.

"Have you ever visited that office?" I inquired.

"No, I haven't," he admitted.

I convinced him that a visit to that office was in order. In fact, it was a *must*. We called, asked if we could come by, and were enthusiastically invited to do so later that afternoon.

The contrast in the two offices was immediately obvious. The layout of this office, the color scheme, the lighting, the fresh flowers, the state-of-the-art equipment, the soft music wafting through the office, the artwork, the friendliness of everyone, and the upscale dispensing area were *spectacular*!

When we left a while later, the optometrist who accompanied me confided, "I now know what my problem is."

In the words of educator John Dewey, "*A problem well-stated is half-solved.*"

More Potential Threats to Think about.

- If your practice currently has little if any "competition" as such, how would you respond if a major optical chain opened across the street?
- What socioeconomic or demographic shifts are occurring in the community that have (or will have) an impact on your practice?
- What are the greatest challenges facing your practice over the next few years that must be overcome to ensure your continued success?
- What would happen if your practice dropped low-paying managed-care plans, or perhaps opted completely out of managed care?

FROM THE SUCCESS FILES

- At one time, Nick Despotidis, O.D., and his partner in Hamilton Square, NJ, accepted approximately 25 different managed-care plans. "We found ourselves practicing in a way that we didn't want to," he says. "We were spending less and less time with each patient. This wasn't the way we built this practice, and it wasn't any fun." As a result, they winnowed out the less-profitable managed-care plans. "Our patient volume dropped by 10%," says Dr. Despotidis, "but in time, the gross increased 7% and our net grew by 25%."[4]
- "Consider the case of John Leeth, O.D., Waynesboro, VA, whose practice was 60% managed care," says consultant Gary Gerber, O.D., Hawthorne, NJ. "Careful analysis of his per-patient revenue revealed that most of his net income came from the 40% who were

private-pay patients. He dropped all managed-care plans and hasn't looked back since. He's increased his net while working a lot less."[5]

- After a seminar I recently conducted in Seattle, WA, Alan Homestead, O.D., wrote, "Your suggestion to drop low-paying insurance plans was interesting. I dropped three plans on January 1, 2000. That was approximately 35% of my patients. However, at the same time I raised my fees. As a result, I am seeing 15% fewer patients and have a 12% increase in revenue this year."

I have heard similar stories from physicians, dentists, podiatrists, psychologists, and other health care providers who have dropped low-paying managed-care plans or opted completely out of managed care.

37 Hard-learned lessons about long-range strategic planning

- "Many practices don't grow because the doctor is so busy examining patients," says Neil B. Gailmard, O.D., M.B.A., F.A.A.O., Munster, IN.
- "Being busy isn't a badge of honor," says Leonard J. Press, O.D., F.A.A.O., F.C.V.D., Fair Lawn, NJ. "It's a badge of stupidity."

Make sure that staff members are involved in the S.W.O.T. analysis. Called *participative management*, this group effort fosters commitment, team spirit, and practice growth.

The S.W.O.T. analysis should lead to a discussion of *focus*, including such additional questions as the following:

- What are the three most important aspects of the practice that require *excellence* to maintain the future growth of the practice?
- What are the most important *changes* we must make this year in order to achieve our goals?

REALITY CHECK

Long-range planning is the key to turning the dreams for your practice into reality. It provides the mechanism to coordinate and focus the activities of day-to-day practice, identifies the most important priorities, and ensures that everyone is rowing in the same direction.

There is no magic formula for strategic planning. If you were to ask 10 management consultants, you'd probably get 10 different methods, all variations on the same theme. The truth is that planning isn't an exact science, and the technique is less important than the process itself.

When we divide seminar audiences into small discussion groups (by practice) and get them started with long-range strategic planning, the excitement builds. Before long, everyone is animated and participating. Sparks fly. One idea acts as a springboard for others, and creative thinking is stimulated. Lists are started of the changes needed, projects, and goals. The high-performance practice is set in motion.

Notes

1. Schmidt EE. Rx for Success. *Optometric Management*, August 2001, 12–13.
2. Hubbs L. Viewpoint. *Optometric Management*, April 2001, 6.
3. Ramsey WS. Extending Your Reach. *Optometric Management*, September 2001, 12–13.
4. Lee J. How to Give Third-Party Plans the Ax. *Review of Optometry*, June 1999.
5. Gerber G. Take It to the Limit. *Review of Optometry*, January 2001, 29.

3

Major Opportunities for Revenue Enhancement and Practice Growth

The American Optometric Association's Workforce Study, conducted by Abt Associates, "alludes to the significant expansion in optometry's scope of practice in recent years with continued increases in patient volume expected in the future. The growth and aging of the population along with growth of managed care will all contribute to this increase."[1]

Opportunities (in the S.W.O.T. analysis) refer to various options for revenue enhancement and practice growth. Consider, for example, the following matrix representing four possibilities:

	Current Services	New Services
Current Patients	1	2
New Patients	3	4

The easiest of the four is No. 1: Getting more of your *current patients* to seek more of your *current services* or purchase more in the optical segment of the practice. It requires nothing new except improved communication skills.

The hardest of the four is No. 4: Acquiring *new patients* for *new services*. In this case, you need to acquire expertise *and* new patients.

Let's start with the easiest.

Strategy No. 1: Current Patients/Current Services

There are many opportunities within this category, including the following:

• Improve acceptance of periodic comprehensive eye examinations

- Activate inactive patients
- Convert "telephone shoppers" into patients
- Increase patient acceptance of premium lens options
- Ask, don't tell
- Prescribe for occupational and avocational vision needs
- The hidden market for quality sunwear
- Tap unused employee health benefits
- Database marketing

38 Improve patient acceptance of periodic comprehensive eye examinations

Two main reasons other than cost that patients don't make appointments to have comprehensive eye examinations are the following:

Lack of information: Some patients believe the only reason to return to an optometrist is for "new glasses." And, if they are seeing fine, there's no reason to return.

Inertia: Many patients know they should periodically have a comprehensive eye examination but never seem to get around to doing it.

Fortunately, both of these problems are manageable.

ACTION STEP

To start, it's essential that patients have a better, more compelling reason than "new glasses" to return to your office for a comprehensive exam. The best, most logical person to provide this reason is the doctor, and the best time to do it is at the end of the exam.

FROM THE SUCCESS FILES

"Whenever we finish examining patients," says Donna Higgins, O.D., Prairie du Chien, WI, "we have reasons for deciding when they should be recalled. We know what we'll be watching for. Don't assume patients also know, without an explanation. You have valid reasons for recommending routine examinations, reasons that are in the patients' best interests. It's simple enough to share those reasons with them."[2]

"When the patient's history is being taken by either the staff or the doctor," says practice management authority Irving Bennett, O.D., "and the patient reveals some systemic condition or disease that has ocular manifestations, the patient should be advised about the need for regular routine care on a semiannual or annual basis, or whatever the problem requires. Diabetes is a good case in point and so is the situation when the patient is taking certain medications. In both these instances, regular monitoring of the retina or of the eye should be done. Patients need to be made aware of this necessity. There is a multitude of eye conditions and systemic diseases that deserve vigilance on the part of an eye care practitioner."[3]

One could make a case that a *failure* to make these recommendations is a *disservice* to the patient—the equivalent of *supervised neglect.*

RECOMMENDED RESOURCE

Vision Council of America, (703) 548-4560, http://www.checkyearly.com

39 Part 2: The recall

After your explanation of why and when a patient should return for a comprehensive eye exam, there are two well-known methods of placing the patient in a recall system:

- Pre-appoint the patient
- Ask the patient's permission to place him or her in the office recall system

"The message of the next yearly examination begins with the doctor," says consultant Barbara Schroer. "The second reminder comes from the business staff during checkout time. The third and fourth messages come from the postcard reminder and the phone call."[4]

FROM THE SUCCESS FILES

"We ask patients if they'd rather we remind them to make an appointment by mail or if they'd like to schedule their next visit at the present time," says Neil B. Gailmard, O.D., M.B.A., F.A.A.O., Munster, IL. "We then do whatever they prefer. The vast majority prefers mail reminders for long-term, routine care."[5]

REALITY CHECK

"If the patient isn't receptive to your explanation while he's sitting in the exam chair," says Jerry Hayes, O.D., Director of the Center for Practice Excellence, "then a postcard or a phone call isn't going to turn him around in 12 months later, either."[6]

Or, as Yogi Berra once said about a slumping ball club playing to empty seats, "If the fans don't want to come to the stadium, there's no way you can stop them."

40 Activate inactive patients

Of all the opportunities for practice growth, none is more logical (or easier) than getting patients who haven't been to the office in 1.5 years (or 2 or even 3 years) to return for a comprehensive eye examination.

ACTION STEPS

To determine its potential, have a staff member call 25 randomly selected "inactive" patients and simply explain the following:

"In reviewing our records, I see that you have not had a comprehensive eye examination since (date). I'm calling to see if you would like to make an appointment at this time."

That's it! No long explanation of *why* it is important, and no reminder that vision anomalies and ocular disease can be present before noticeable symptoms arise. Certainly, use no scare tactics, sales pitch, or "inducements" of any kind. Have your staff member keep everything low-key, and see what the patient says.

Your staff member may learn the patient has moved away or because of managed care or some other reason is seeing another optometrist. Or the patient may say, "I'm doing fine and don't care to make an appointment at this time."

Let's just focus on what many receptionists have found to be a surprising number of patients who say one of the following:

- "Has it really been that long?" (2 years?)
- "I know it's been a long time. I've been meaning to call you."

- "I've been waiting for you to call me."

Needless to say, any one of these replies will lead to an appointment.

Tested Tip.   After making the appointment, have your staff member ask the patient, "Is there anyone else in your family for whom you'd like to make an appointment?" Again, there'll be more "yes" answers than you might guess.

Make sure, however, the staff member making such calls is "comfortable" doing it and truly believes it's in the patient's best interests—he or she will get better results.

A handful of favorable responses more than warrants telephoning the balance of your inactive patients.

FROM THE SUCCESS FILES

"Cherry-pick certain charts to increase your odds of success," recommends Gary Gerber, O.D., Hawthorne, NJ. "For example, pull old files of patients who dropped out of contact lenses because they had problems with lens deposits. Offer them a free consultation to determine if daily disposables are right for them. Similarly, offer dry eye patients a free consultation to see if punctal occlusion will work."[7]

BENCHMARK

Caring for the Eyes of America 2002, published by the American Optometric Association, reports that in 2001, the median interval between comprehensive eye examinations (including refractions) for established patients was 16.5 months.[8]

41 Avoid these tactics

The following are examples of what patients in focus groups have interpreted as "high-pressure tactics" when called by optometric office personnel to schedule an appointment:

- Continuing to talk after the patient says, "You've caught me at a bad time. . ." (and then telling the patient, "This will only take a minute. . .").

- Giving the patient a long explanation of why an exam is important (the time for that was at the end of the exam, as previously explained).
- Putting patients on the defensive when they show no interest in making an appointment by asking, for example, their reasons for not doing so. (Employee incentive plans are often the motivating factor in such situations.)
- Asking the patient to make an appointment by offering a choice of two appointment times (e.g., Monday at 10:30 or Thursday at 3:30). That is an old, very recognizable form of high pressure and is resented by many patients.
- Being too persistent with follow-up calls. (*Better approach*: ask patients if they would like to be called again in 30 or 60 days. If patients say, "I'll call you back," don't press the issue. Simply say, "That will be fine.")

ACID TEST

A high percentage of "no shows" for such appointments might indicate that the person making the calls is using more high pressure than he/she may realize (or intends), and patients only agree to make appointments to get off the phone.

42 Convert "telephone shoppers" into patients

Some staff members think of "telephone shoppers" as *nuisance calls*. Two or three such calls a week are not uncommon in some offices. Others receive that many or more in a single day. Properly handled, many of these callers become patients.

REALITY CHECK

If you are satisfied with the percentage of "telephone shoppers" who make and keep appointments, do not change a thing. If you think there may be room for improvement, however, have your front desk personnel try the following protocol—it's been used with success by many offices.

ACTION STEPS

If callers are asking, for example, about the cost of an examination, eyewear, contact lenses, or vision therapy, give them an answer. Refusal to do so may strike some as unreasonable, if not suspicious. And, for people who simply want to know if they have enough cash on hand to cover the expense, it's downright silly.

In her training guide, *Telephone Skills That Build Business*, Terry Theiss, C.P.O.T., A.B.O.C., suggests quoting fees "as a range, as an average, or as the lowest possible fee."[9]

"Patients call up and ask how much contact lenses cost," says Gregg Ossip, O.D., Indianapolis, IN. "That's not really the question they want to ask, but it's the only question they know. The majority of offices simply say, 'Contact lenses cost X dollars.'

"Instead, we interview them over the phone to determine their needs. We describe our examination, which includes topography, retinal photographs, autorefraction, autokeratometry, and screening fields. We say, 'Come in, we'll give you an honest opinion of what options are open to you.' We're not trying to sell over the telephone, which is very, very hard to do."[10]

Tested Tip. Consider asking callers if they're "shopping," and if so, suggest they make sure the fees quoted elsewhere are "all inclusive" (if that's the way your fees are quoted). Then, explain in more detail: It eliminates the confusion caused by "low ball" quotes from other offices.

"Discount providers (of LASIK surgery) are confusing the public on price," says Jeffrey Augustine, O.D., Center Director for Clear Choice Laser Centers in Brecksville, OH. In his view, the discounters are actually offering à la carte refractive surgery by advertising a lower price for just the surgical procedure, then charging separately for additional services that are essential for the overall success of the entire procedure.[11]

Next, offer to send telephone shoppers a practice brochure or refer them to your Web site.

Tested Tip. Photographs, impressive credentials, and an overview of your office, presented in an attractive practice brochure or user-friendly Web site, help discerning, quality-oriented patients to decide in your favor, regardless of fees.

Last, call a few days later to ask if the patient received the brochure or had an opportunity to view the Web site. If so, are there any questions? If not, would he or she like to make an appointment?

Tested Tip.   If the person is undecided, consider offering a brief, no-charge visit if meeting the doctor and seeing the office would be helpful.

---

43 Increase patient acceptance of premium lens options

Premium lens options such as antireflective coating, ultraviolet (UV) protection, high-index materials, progressive addition lenses, polished edges, and the like, greatly improve a patient's visual efficiency, comfort, safety, and appearance. That's a given.

FROM THE SUCCESS FILES

The following are some proven ways to increase patient acceptance of these options:

Begin in the Exam Room.   "When you discuss products in the exam room," says Michael H. Cho, O.D., F.A.A.O., Director of Optical Services at the University of Alabama at Birmingham School of Optometry, "patients interpret what you say as a prescription or recommendation. This also paves the way for you to properly transfer authority to your staff. For example, when I recommend a specific PAL in high index with an antireflective coating, I tell the patient that the optometric assistant or optician will discuss and answer any questions about these products in depth. By doing this, I've integrated products with services, transferred authority, motivated the patient to visit our dispensary, and set a proactive example for the staff to follow."[12]

This all-important *transfer of authority* can also be accomplished by escorting the patient to the dispensary, or by calling the optician into the exam room and, in each case, reviewing the premium lens recommendations in front of the patient.

Point Out the Medical Benefits.   "You may have mentioned that UV protection cuts down on glare," says John H. McDougall, O.D., Quincy, IL, "but don't forget to mention the option's main benefit.

Tell the patient, 'UV rays are potentially harmful to the eye, and this is a special concern now that the ozone layer is being depleted. Just as dermatologists warn you to wear sunscreen if you're outside a lot, I recommend that you put UV protection in your glasses.'"[13]

HARD-LEARNED LESSON

Do not present people with solutions to problems until they understand the problems.

It Is Your Duty to Warn. "Any patient can benefit from the impact resistance and lightweight characteristics of polycarbonate," says Robert J. Lee, O.D., Cerritos, CA. "But for some patients, these characteristics are more than just a convenience. If a patient is monocular or has the potential for eye injury because of involvement in sports, job or hobby-related hazards, or simply because he or she is a child, make sure you discuss the impact-resistant properties of polycarbonate."*[14]

"If a patient refuses to accept your recommendation for polycarbonate," says Pamela J. Miller, O.D., J.D., Highland, CA, "be certain you document that fact. The following is the form we use:"[15]

I understand that my doctor has recommended the following for my safety and protection. I am aware of the advantages and disadvantages of this recommendation and have decided to select a different option.

Date_____   Recommendation_____

Reason_____

Signed_____
          (Patient, Parent, Guardian)

"When we started asking people to sign off that they had declined polycarbonate lenses," says Texas Smith, O.D., Citrus Heights, CA, "our sales went through the roof. Today, we do over 70% in poly. It was all because of this disclaimer for 'Duty to Warn.'"[16]

---

*Recently, a new ophthalmic lens material with impact-resistant characteristics similar to polycarbonate has been introduced under the trade name Trivex.

RECOMMENDED RESOURCES

Polycarbonate Lens Council, (800) 944-6206, http://www.polycarb.org
Duty to Warn Kit available from Optical Laboratories Association, (800) 477-5652, http://www.ola-labs.org

Discuss Lenses First. "In many parts of Europe, it's lenses that are presented first," says Stephanie K. De Long, Editor-in-Chief of *Eyecare Business*. "That serves several purposes. It puts the emphasis on the optician's expertise. It underscores the importance and value of technology. And it helps the optician retain control of the dispensing situation."[17]

FROM THE SUCCESS FILES

"It is good practice," writes Neil Gailmard, O.D. F.A.A.O., Munster, IN, "to begin the dispensing visit with a discussion of the lenses, before frames are considered, perhaps at an in-office 'lens design center.' This special area is devoted to samples and demonstration lenses in the form of uncut lens blanks (e.g., high-index plastic vs. CR-39 in the same prescription) and mockup glasses (e.g., right lens antireflective coat, left lens normal)."[18]

Bundle Fees. "Quote fees as one package instead of a series of add-ons," says Robert J. Lee, O.D., Cerritos, CA. "Presenting features as a series of add-ons emphasizes costs over benefits and invites patients to compromise. If a patient balks at the cost, inquire which feature(s) the patient doesn't want. Then you can remove options and quote the total fee again."[19]

Stress the Benefits of Premium Lens Options. For example, "Antireflective coating isn't just for making glasses look good," says Irving Bennett, O.D., founder of the Irving Bennett Business and Practice Management Center at the Pennsylvania College of Optometry. "It improves night vision, a major advantage for senior patients. Progressive lenses aren't just to get rid of unsightly bifocal lines. They provide major improvements in vision at all ranges."[20]

RECOMMENDED RESOURCE

The Antireflective Council of America, (877) 254-4477, http://www.arcouncil.org

Make Sure You and Your Staff "Walk Your Talk." "If you recommend antireflection verbally, but don't wear it yourself," says Gary Heiting, O.D., Hopkins, MN, "the patient receives conflicting messages and is more likely to believe the more powerful nonverbal message."[21]

ACTION STEP

Give patients a chance to say "no" to premium lens options that will improve their visual efficiency, comfort, safety, and appearance, but don't be overbearing. Avoid the "hard sell." Don't sacrifice long-term relationships for short-term profits.

44 Ask, don't tell

Get patients involved with discovering their vision needs by asking questions such as the following:

- Ask bifocal wearers if they ever watch television from a *recliner chair.* If the answer is *yes*, ask: "Does the bifocal portion get in your line of vision? Cause neck strain? Do you ever slide your glasses down your nose so you can see more easily through the distance portion?" If so, suggest the patient have his or her distance prescription mounted in any old frame at home and keep it by the TV. Comfort is important and patients will be delighted with their "TV glasses." It's an idea I first heard about from Douglas D. McElfresh, O.D., San Diego, CA.
- Ask presbyopic golfers if their bifocal gets in the way of their swing. If "yes," ask if they've ever seen a special lens just for golf. Then, show them a pair of "golf glasses" with a 10-mm button seg in the temporal, lower corner of the right lens only (for a right-handed golfer). It gives them an unobstructed view of the ball, does not interfere with their swing, and yet is fine for writing the score.

Golfers will love the convenience of not taking their glasses on and off, *plus* this unusual prescription will likely generate some conversation among their golfing partners, and possibly referrals.

In our surveys, only a handful of golfers had ever *heard* of such an idea, let alone been *asked* if they would like it. Most said it sounded like a great idea and asked where they could get such lenses.

- Ask patients if they're bothered by the weight or thickness of their lenses, by bright sunlight, by the line of their bifocal, or by glare or reflections when using a computer or driving at night. Ask patients if they (or their children) engage in sports in which *eye safety* is a factor.

You'll get both "yes" and "no" answers. Don't be surprised though, if patients have never thought about these problems. By raising the issue, you will "plant the seed," causing them to think about the weight of their lenses and how often they push their glasses up, or whether they're bothered by glare or the line of a bifocal. Before long, some will return for premium lenses—I've seen it happen countless times.

REALITY CHECK

The reason that more premium and special-purpose lenses aren't dispensed isn't because of the cost or lack of interest—but rather because they're not shown and explained to patients.

HARD-LEARNED LESSON

"Give patients the chance to think about contact lenses during the entire time in your office," says Gary Gerber, O.D., Hawthorn, NJ, "instead of waiting until the last possible moment when they are already focused on leaving the office. You've often read that a way to build your contact lens practice is to ask patients, 'Have you ever thought about contact lenses?' It's a good question—and asking it sooner is better than asking it later."[22]

"Do more than fit spherical myopes with 2-week disposable contacts on a daily wear basis," says Carmen Castellano, O.D., St. Louis, MO. "Instead, routinely fit mild-to-moderate astigmats with soft toric lenses and don't be afraid to recommend contact lenses to high or oblique astigmats. Don't shy away from extended wear where indicated, and fit many presbyopes. You'll find your percentage of rigid gas-permeable wearers to be much higher than the 15% national average."[23]

A Related Idea. "Your patient information sheet should include a line that asks if patients would be interested in contact lenses that change eye color," say Janice M. Jurkus, O.D., M.B.A., and Jeffrey Sonsino, O.D. "Fitting can then be streamlined to the specific lens type you deem best for the patient. If your support staff members wear contact lenses, suggest they wear tinted ones. Patients who see different colored lenses on real people (rather than in pictures) are more likely to ask about availability."[24]

HARD-LEARNED LESSON

Our surveys indicate that significantly more tinted contact lenses are dispensed in offices in which *staff members wear the lenses* than in offices in which they don't.

45 Prescribe for occupational and avocational vision needs

Some practitioners use an entrance history form that asks patients about their occupations, hobbies, and sports interests to ascertain their vision needs. Others include such questions during the case history.

The VDT Workplace Questionnaire, recommended by Jeffrey Anshel, B.S., O.D., Encinitas, CA, includes questions about work practices, the environment (including the lighting), display screen, workstation (including viewing distances), and visual symptoms. Even the most unlikely candidates, he points out, are often avid Internet users.

"By asking the right questions and performing the appropriate tests," says Dr. Anshel, "we gain insight into the patient's daily vision use."[25]

Diagnosing patients' occupational and avocational vision needs is the first step. The next is to *prescribe* special-purpose lenses and/or premium lens options that then provide optimum visual performance.

This in-depth consideration of patients' total vision needs benefits your practice in several ways: It provides a unique, value-added service to patients, differentiates your practice, and generates significant additional revenue.

46 Hidden market for quality sunwear

Patients often buy ready-made sunglasses of poor quality at drug or department stores, and, sometimes, street vendors. Yet, unless they experience serious discomfort, most patients would not think of bringing such sunglasses to your office. Some would see no reason to do so, and others would be embarrassed to do so.

ACTION STEPS

Provide a value-added service to such patients that also has the potential to generate considerable additional revenue:

When making appointments, have your receptionist suggest that patients bring in any sunglasses they are currently using, regardless of where they were obtained. The purpose? "To make sure you have clear, comfortable vision with them, are protected properly from the harmful rays of the sun, and have a frame that fits properly and is comfortable." The gesture alone will be appreciated.

During the examination, place the sunglasses over the aperture of the acuity projector to determine if there is unwanted power or distortion in the lenses. Check for visible light, infrared, and UV transmittance. The fit of the frame should also be checked.

Many over-the-counter sunglasses are fine. Others are seriously flawed. When such shortcomings are explained and demonstrated to patients, many want quality sunwear replacements.

REALITY CHECK

Failure to evaluate potentially harmful sunglasses is a disservice to patients. It's also a lost opportunity.

FROM THE SUCCESS FILES

"Education is the key to sunglasses success for contact lens patients," says Sheila Wood, O.D., Washington, DC, who estimates that 65–75% of her contact lens patients now have sunglasses.[26]

47 Tap unused employee health benefits

Many employer-based health benefit packages provide vision care benefits that must be used in the course of a calendar year.

FROM THE SUCCESS FILES

"Many patients simply forget to use health plan benefits during the course of the year," says Richard Edlow, O.D., Baltimore, MD. "As a result, they enter into the final months of each year with benefits they must essentially use or lose. We can do our patients a great service," he adds, "by reminding them to take advantage of any unused health plan benefits before year's end."[27]

ACTION STEP

October through November is a good time to remind insurance and third-party patients of the unused vision care benefits available to them. Post notices on the practice Web site or include them on monthly statements. E-mail is another alternative (see next item). Practitioners who do so invariably have a busier-than-usual December.

48 Database marketing

This opportunity for revenue enhancement and practice growth involves searching your database of patients and then sending informative mailings to those that fit a certain profile.

FROM THE SUCCESS FILES

Before the allergy season begins, Morris F. Sheffer, O.D., Charlotte, NC, uses that database to identify patients who suffer from allergic conjunctivitis and giant papillary conjunctivitis. He then sends letters to these patients advising them to schedule appointments before their symptoms start. He also informs them when a new medication becomes available that relieves the symptoms of allergy and, more importantly, may prevent the symptoms.[28]

"This allergy season," he told me, "we mailed 175 letters to allergy sufferers who had been in the previous season with conjunctivitis. Approximately 45 patients responded by coming in for an eye exam or office visit."

"While most practitioners give patients the option to contact the practice via e-mail through the practice Web site," says Barbara Anan Kogan, O.D., "outgoing e-mail is still largely overlooked as a patient retention and recall tool. With a growing number of patients having e-mail addresses, e-mail has become an excellent way to contact patients for 6-month contact lens evaluations, 3-month glaucoma follow-ups, diabetic retinopathy care, vision therapy sessions, or simply annual examinations."[29]

ACTION STEP

Make sure there is a place for the patient's e-mail address on your patient information form and also that you have your e-mail and Web site addresses on your letterhead and the business cards of you and your staff.

This is only a sampling of many possible strategies to interest current patients in more of your current services and products.

Strategies No. 2 and No. 4: Add New Services

The following are some of the many ways that new services can contribute to revenue enhancement and practice growth.

49 Sports vision services

"You can provide a wide range of (sports vision) services," says Alan Berman, O.D., who is co-director of the Institute for Sports Vision (along with Donald S. Teig, O.D., and Geoffrey Heddle, O.D.) in Ridgefield, CT. "We provide anything from protective eyewear to sport-specific contact lenses to evaluation of how the eyes are performing on the field. We test eye muscle function, eye-hand coordination, peripheral vision, and reaction time."[30]

50 Nursing home services

"I have a private practice but also spend 30% of my week in nursing home facilities," says Noah M. Eger, O.D., F.A.A.O., Coraopolis, PA. "This niche has provided me the opportunity to help many whose eyes have long been neglected. By making these patients more comfortable and improving their vision, it lets them become more active and enjoy a better quality of life. At the same time, my private practice has grown in large part to my nursing home practice. Physicians, nurses, staff, and family members appreciate my services and travel to my office for their eye care."[31]

RECOMMENDED RESOURCE

Optometric Care of Nursing Home Residents (Published by the American Optometric Association), 1998.

51 Therapeutic services

"Adding therapeutics to my practice has helped us most to concentrate on the medical aspects of optometry," says Phillip E. Apfel, O.D., Cincinnati, OH. "For example, our glaucoma patients, who are mainly covered by third-party payers, are a constant source of income, along with their referrals. Co-managing refractive surgery patients, as well as treating dry eye patients with collagen and punctal plugs, has also been a steady source of income during difficult economic times."[32]

52   Dry eye therapy

"Dry eye therapy represents the biggest growth opportunity for most practices," says Arthur B. Epstein, O.D., F.A.A.O., Roslyn, NY. "However, many eye care practitioners have virtually ignored this area. As America grays, the prevalence of dry eye increases."[33]

53   Traditional optometry

"Clearly, optometry is moving towards more therapeutics," says Walter S. Ramsey, O.D., F.A.A.O., Charleston, WV. "But don't neglect the dispensing end of your profession. These fees provide the greatest potential for profit margin. My practice had become too heavily involved in therapeutics. In an average month, it wasn't unusual for pathology-related visits to account for more than 40% of patient encounters. I knew from an economic standpoint I should redirect more attention toward traditional optometry to capture more optical business and bring my practice back into balance."[34]

HARD-LEARNED LESSON

"We strayed from what got us to the top of the mountain, and it cost us greatly" (William Clay Ford, CEO, Ford Motor Co.).

54   Multifocal contact lenses

The hottest untapped market today, says Mary Jo Stiegmeier, O.D., Beachwood, OH, is fitting presbyopes with multifocal contact lenses. "There's a multitude of new and diverse bifocal, multifocal and progressive contact lenses available in soft, disposable, soft toric, and gas permeable options." She adds, "Satisfy a presbyopic contact lens wearer, and you'll see your referrals climb through the roof."[35]

55 Low vision services

Eyecare Business recently conducted a survey of optometrists who added low vision to their practices during the past 5 years (as opposed to those who specialize in low vision). The majority (62%) of those surveyed say they did it to differentiate or grow their practices. Another 18% were motivated primarily by the potential income that the pent-up demand for low vision services could produce, and 12% said they considered low vision their ethical obligation.[36]

Strategies No. 3 and No. 4: Attract New Patients

New patients, by definition, offer limitless opportunities for revenue enhancement and practice growth. Here are some of the options:

56 Join third-party plans

The 20/20 Managed Vision Care Survey 1999 found that, among surveyed optometrists, 50.3% said managed care had increased their patient base; 9.9% reported a decrease. What effect did managed care have on overall practice revenues? 29.8% of doctors of optometry reported an increase, 27.6% reported a decrease, and 42.5% said their overall practice revenues were the same.[37]

REALITY CHECK

"Signing up with plans to increase patient volume and fill excess capacity is one thing," caution consultants Gil Weber and Alan H. Cleinman. "But, if signing onto a plan pushes better paying patients out of appointment slots, that makes no business sense, especially if it also increases administrative costs and strips away margins. Furthermore, plans which motivate the delivery, directly or indirectly, of a different level of service to one patient versus another are to be avoided at all cost."[38]

HARD-LEARNED LESSON

Do not expect that managed-care patients will refer private pay patients. Managed-care patients typically refer more managed-care patients.

57 Attract more private pay patients

"To attract and keep patients who are willing to pay out of pocket for vision care," says Judith Lee, Senior Contributing Editor to *Review of Optometry*, "treat patients better. You may think you already treat them great, but go several steps further. Private-pay patients will choose an environment that makes them feel special. Think about patient comfort: Offer coffee and soft drinks, let them use the phone, give them a place to plug in a laptop, and provide videos for kids. Give them stuff, such as lens solutions or nice eyeglass cases."[39]

"In order to attract private-pay patients," says Russell G. Rosenquist, D.D.S., Glenview, IL, and past president of the American Academy of Dental Practice Administration, "you must:

- Have high-level clinical competency and an office that runs smoothly and efficiently.
- Have a physical facility that is convenient, modern, and noticeably clean (not just clean, but *noticeably* clean).
- Have a team that are outgoing, well groomed, dressed professionally; has great smiles; love people; and is well trained for their respective jobs. In addition, the respect between the doctor and staff must be obvious.
- Have a local study club with whom you can talk about practice-related problems and share confidences.
- Build the patient's confidence and trust in you. *Earned trust* is the key to patient acceptance and loyalty.

- Give patients an easy-to-understand reason to return for periodic maintenance visits and then pre-appoint them. More than 90% will comply.
- Don't be afraid to ask for referrals. "The phrase with which I'm comfortable," Dr. Rosenquist says, "is 'We need and appreciate your referral of friends to our office.' Start saying that to patients and you may be surprised to have them reply, 'I didn't realize you were taking new patients.'"

Note: There are countless additional ideas throughout this book for attracting new patients, private-pay or otherwise, and equally important, for *keeping them* in your practice.

REALITY CHECK

If what you are doing in your independent, fee-for-service practice is no better, no different, or perceived to be no better or different than what's being done in managed-care offices, then what incentive do patients have to remain in your practice?

58 Yellow Pages advertising? Read this first

Most optometrists who advertise in the Yellow Pages are doing so to attract new patients, perhaps jump-start a new or sluggish practice, or replace patients lost to a managed-care plan to which they don't belong. Is such advertising a good investment?

The consensus of optometrists I've surveyed at seminars throughout the country is that Yellow Pages advertising is of limited value in attracting new patients.

REALITY CHECK

Caring for the Eyes of America 2002, published by the American Optometric Association, reported that, in 2001, the percentage of consumers finding an eye doctor through the Yellow Pages was only 5.8%.[8]

Similar statistics are found in other healthcare professions. Edwin D. Secord, D.D.S., past President of the Detroit District Dental Society, writing in the *Detroit Dental Bulletin*, put it this way: "Where do my best patients come from? They come from present patients, referring dentists, and personal friends. Where do my worst patients come from? The Yellow Pages. There are exceptions, but this generally holds true."

Optometrists who purchase bold listings and varying sized display ads in their local telephone Yellow Pages often discover (too late) that their ads are completely overshadowed by larger, more attention-getting ads of other optometric practices and optical chains, greatly reducing the effectiveness of their ads.

In addition, optometrists who track the response to their Yellow Pages advertising report that in many cases, the low numbers of new patients simply do not warrant the cost of the ads. As a result, many O.D.s have discontinued Yellow Pages advertising with little, if any, drop in the number of new patients they are seeing.

The Park Avenue (New York) office of Andrea Thau, O.D., president of the New York State Optometric Association, has *no* Yellow Pages listing—none at all, and no "outdoor sign" except for a small brass plaque on the exterior of the building—yet her primary care practice continues to grow (three doctors of optometry, soon to be four). How? By word-of-mouth.

REALITY CHECK

To determine if such advertising has been a good investment for your practice, include the following question on the Patient Information Form that new patients fill out on their first visit:

How did you first hear about our practice?

Then, give patients a choice, such as an outdoor sign, directory provided by an insurance company, phone book, physician, or personal recommendation. Consider also, including after personal recommendation, the question, "Whom may we thank for referring you?"

Key Words Used in This Survey.

- The word *first* in the initial question is critical. Oddly enough, some patients say they first learned about the practice from the phone book, when in fact, it was only where they obtained your address and telephone number. With further probing, you or a staff member may find they *first* heard about your practice from a friend, co-worker, physician, pharmacist, or the emergency room at the local hospital, and *then* looked in the phone book.

- In most cases, patients have freedom of choice when given a directory of providers by an insurance company or managed-care plan. Many patients seeing your name will *still ask* someone's opinion before selecting your office.

- A small but significant point: The word "refer" (as in "Whom may we thank for referring you?") is associated in some patients' minds with a *doctor's* referral. In such cases, when it was a *friend* (not a doctor) who told them about the practice, they often leave the answer blank. Thus, the preferred wording for the Patient Information Form is "Whom may we thank for *telling* you about our practice?"

ACTION STEPS

Survey new patients for the next 90 days and then do the math. If the return on your advertising is worth it, take a bigger ad. If not, put those dollars to work in a way that achieves better return on investment.

---

59 Is your busy practice sending the wrong message?

"Nothing succeeds like success," goes the old saying. And *looking busy* does say you're successful. In fact, it's a great image! If your "busy-ness" looks *excessive,* however, it can send the wrong message—antagonizing patients and discouraging referrals.

An example of such overkill: optometrists who are always behind schedule and "complain" (perhaps "brag") how *swamped* they are. They come across as breathless and time pressured. It may be true, but it's the wrong message to send to patients who are paying for your time and expertise and expect someone who is alert, attentive, and at his or her best.

ACTION STEP

If your practice is truly that busy, hire additional full-time or part-time employees to shoulder some of the work. If, for example, the front desk is so harried that people are frequently put on hold, often for a long time, and when finally connected, are *rushed*, then get extra help at the front desk, if only for the "peak periods." Or, if you're the one who is harried and often rushed to stay on schedule, delegate some of what you do to others, or hire an associate. Most important: When telling patients, physicians, and other referral sources how busy your practice is, stop short of making it sound as if you are too busy to see new patients or give existing patients the time and attention to which they're entitled. Beware especially of complaints to patients about the avalanche of patients created by managed care. The same is true for your staff.

REALITY CHECK

Are you or your staff members ever asked if you're taking new patients? If so, do some marketing research by replying, "Yes, we are, but what makes you ask?" You may learn that your practice is indeed sending the wrong message.

NETWORKING

Of all the strategies for attracting new patients, private pay or otherwise, *networking* can be one of the most rewarding and personally satisfying. Because of its importance, the next chapter has been devoted to it.

Notes

1. Workforce Study Shows ODs Expanding Market Share, Capacity to Serve Unmet Needs. *AOA News*, February 14, 2000, 1,4.
2. Higgins D. Encouraging Patients to Understand the Rationale for Routine Examination. *Optometric Management*, March 2001, 89–92.
3. Bennett I. *Management for the Eye Care Practitioner*. Butterworth–Heinemann, 1993, 92.
4. Schroer B. Now Is the Time to Plan Your Strategy for Next Year. *Primary Care Optometry News*, December 1996, 14–15.
5. Gailmard NB. Is Preappointing the Best Recall Method? *Optometric Management*, November 2000, 81,111.
6. Hayes J. Total Recall. *Optometric Management*, September 2000, 24.
7. Gerber G. Thar's Gold in Thar Files. *Review of Optometry*, April 1999.
8. *Caring for the Eyes of America 2002*. American Optometric Association, St. Louis, MO, 2002.
9. Theiss T. Telephone Skills That Build Business. *Primary Eyecare Network*, 2001, 31.

10. Using High-End Dispensing Techniques. *Optometric Management*, February 1998, 7S,10S.
11. Rosenthal T. Discount Laser Centers No Match for Today's Co-Managing ODs. *Primary Care Optometry News*, August 2001, 18–19.
12. Cho MH. Increasing Your PALs Prescription Rate. *Optometric Management*, February 1998, 89–90,94.
13. McDougall JH. How to Master the One-Minute Introduction. *Optometric Management*, February 1994, 33–34.
14. Lee RJ. Growing Your Practice with Evolving Lens Technology. *Optometric Management*, October 1997, 87–89.
15. Miller PJ. *A Handbook for the Ophthalmic Practice*. Santa Ana, CA: Optometric Extension Program Foundation, 1997.
16. Morgan E. Doing Your Duty. *Eyecare Business*, July 2001, 88.
17. De Long SK. A Win-Win Strategy for Survival. *Eyecare Business*, 1999, 34–38.
18. Gailmard NB. Ophthalmic Dispensing. *Business Aspects of Optometry*, edited by Classé JG, et al., Boston: Butterworth–Heinemann, 1997, 203–212.
19. Lee RJ. Growing Your Practice with Evolving Lens Technology. *Optometric Management*, October 1997, 87–89,92.
20. Bennett I. A Baker's Dozen of Hot Tips for a New Practice. *New O.D.* supplement to *Optometric Management*, December 1998, 22,24–25.
21. Heiting G. How to Present Anti-Reflective Coatings. *Optometric Management*, March 1998, 3S–8S.
22. Gerber G. First Things First—Mention Contact Lenses to Your Patients. *Contact Lens Spectrum*, November 2001, 48.
23. Castellano C. 14 Ways to Develop and Market Your Contact Lens Practice. *Optometric Management*, January 2002, 55–58.
24. Jurkus JM, Sonsino J. The Many Applications of Tinted Contact Lenses. *Contact Lens Spectrum*, December 2001, 24,26–29.
25. Anshel J. Are You Treating Computer Vision Syndrome Yet? *Optometric Management*, April 2000, 65,68,72,74.
26. Kogan BA. Making the Connection: Contacts and Sunglasses. *Eyecare Business*, March 2000, 151,154,156.
27. Time to Tap Unused Employee Health Benefits. *Optometry*, November 2000, 746.
28. Sheffer MF. Innovating with Internal Marketing. *Optometric Management*, May 1998, 57–58,60.
29. Kogan BA. Practice Strategies. *Optometry*, October 2000, 672.
30. Byrne J. Sports Vision: A Valuable Service for Professional, Amateur Athletes. *Primary Care Optometry News*, December 2001, 20–21.
31. Eger NM. Taking a Closer Look at Nursing Homes. *Optometric Management*, September 1999, 38–44.

32. Apfel PE. Letter to the Editor. *Optometric Management*, May 2001, 8.
33. Epstein AB. Talking TPAs, Four Conversations You Need to Hear. *Optometric Management*, March 1999, 13S.
34. Ramsey WS. Extending Your Reach. *Optometric Management*, September 2001, 12–13.
35. Stiegmeier MJ. Are You Overlooking the Hottest, Untapped Market Today? *Optometric Management*, February 1998, 68–69,71.
36. Focus on Low Vision. A Supplement to *Eyecare Business*, June 2001, 8.
37. Krasnogor E. Market Pulse. *20/20*, March 2000, 122–123.
38. Weber G, Cleinman A. Choosing the Right Managed Care Plans. *Eyecare Business*, October 1999, 40,42,44.
39. Lee J. How to Court Private Payers. *Review of Optometry*, April 2001, 29.

4

Secrets of Savvy Networking

"What's the worst thing you can say about another doctor?" asks otolaryngologist/allergist Martin H. Zwerling, Aiken, SC. "That he's incompetent, lazy, dishonest? No—the worst thing you can say is, 'I never heard of him.' Building your own practice," he adds, "means developing effective relationships with your colleagues in the community."[1]

Networking is one means of getting known and developing effective relationships with colleagues and other health care practitioners. It often leads to sharing of information and reciprocal referrals. These include primary care physicians, ophthalmologists, other optometrists, neurologists, pediatricians, plastic surgeons, pharmacists, psychologists, athletic coaches, occupational therapists, hospital emergency room personnel, school nurses, and teachers, among others.

This chapter describes some of the ways that high-performance optometrists have used networking to forge these relationships.

REALITY CHECK

At the outset, I recognize that the medical marketplace in some cases is *politically driven*, making it extremely difficult to earn physician referrals, even when well deserved. In other cases, the process is *economically driven* by patients who may prefer your services but whose health care plans will not pay for them.

Notwithstanding, countless high-performance optometrists *have* used networking as a strategy for practice growth. Here are some of their secrets:

60 Hospital privileges

"Obtaining hospital privileges may be the most significant thing you can do to receive physician referrals," says James C. Leadingham, O.D., Ashland, KY. "Staff meetings at hospitals give you a reason to regularly meet with family practitioners. This one-to-one relationship is the best possible way to establish a referral relationship."[2]

REALITY CHECK

"Getting hospital privileges in the New York metro area was no easy task," admits Arthur B. Epstein, O.D., F.A.A.O., who today is director of the Contact Lens Service at North Shore University Hospital, New York University School of Medicine, Great Neck, NY. "Once in," he says, "I ran with the ball, spending countless hours teaching contact lens courses while simultaneously taking advantage of the learning experiences that I could not have gotten in private practice. This opportunity still didn't get me anywhere in terms of privileges, which required several years of hard work and proving my value."[3]

RECOMMENDED RESOURCE

Optometric Hospital Privileges (Published by the American Optometric Association [AOA])

61 Volunteer optometric services

Participate in some type of charity program, such as the following:

- Volunteers in Service in Our Nation (VISION) USA is a nonprofit, tax-exempt charity developed by members of the AOA. Its sole purpose is to provide basic eye health and vision care services without charge to individuals who have no other means of obtaining care. VISION USA benefits an estimated 30 million working people and their families in the United States who have low incomes and need eye care but cannot afford insurance or the cost of ordinary care. Because these people work and earn income, they often fall between the gaps of government and private health care assistance programs. For more information, visit http://www. aoanet.org.

- VOSH (Volunteer Optometric Services to Humanity) is an organization of optometrists and other interested individuals who are dedicated to providing vision care to people around the world who cannot afford or obtain it. For further information, contact: VOSH Inc., Box 19028, Indianapolis, IN 46219; http://www.vosh.org.
- Operation Bright Start (OBS) is a network of volunteer doctors committed to early diagnosis, treatment, and prevention of eye and vision disorders among infants in the United States. "We wrote to all physicians, physicians' assistants, nurse practitioners, and anyone in our community who had the potential to see the infant population, and informed them of the (no-charge) service we provide," says W. David Sullins Jr., O.D., Athens, TN, former AOA president and chairman of OBS. "Additionally, we sent copies of the OBS assessment to the patient's primary care providers. In time, Woods Memorial Hospital in Etowah, TN, asked if it could distribute the pamphlets detailing OBS to birthing centers, Lamaze classes, and parenting education classes. The concept," says Dr. Sullins, "has been a wonderful experience for our community and our clinic. OBS has enabled us to detect problems early in life and take a preventive role. It has enhanced our relationship with the pediatricians, physicians' assistants, nurse practitioners, and pediatric ophthalmic surgeons in the area as well as local hospitals. And, it has enhanced our reputation and relationship with our community." But even these benefits, adds Dr. Sullins, "fall short of the good feeling you get when you take care of children."[4]

FROM THE SUCCESS FILES

In the last 2 years, Jason Clopton, O.D., Cookeville, TN, has examined more than 200 infants in conjunction with the OBS program. "Approximately 15 had vision problems, including undiagnosed amblyopia and strabismus. After sending reports to the family's physician, the referrals began coming in, not only from physicians, but also from impressed parents. What I didn't anticipate when I started," Dr. Clopton told me, "is the tremendous impact this program would have on my practice."

Further information about OBS is available from the American Foundation for Vision Awareness, 243 N. Lindberg Blvd., St. Louis, MO 63141, (800) 927-AFVA; http://www.afva.org.

Give some thought to these worthwhile programs. In addition to the immense personal satisfaction you'll get from helping those in need, you'll earn tremendous respect from your professional colleagues and the community at large.

62 Co-management of the diabetic patient

"When it comes to caring for diabetic patients," Randolph Brooks, O.D., Ledgewood, NJ, believes, "we are part of a larger team rather than in a league of our own. Communication with each team member makes for a winning game plan in which other doctors know that we provide excellent clinical care and help to achieve a successful outcome. Send report letters about each diabetic patient," he advises, "to his or her primary care physician and copies to any other specialist the patient sees. This is especially important when caring for patients whose blood sugar is poorly controlled or who don't see their GP regularly."[5]

63 Use a common language

Leonard J. Press, O.D., F.C.O.V.D., F.A.A.O., Fair Lawn, NJ, whose specialty is pediatric and adult vision therapy, suggests that the key to networking with pediatricians and pediatric ophthalmologists is to talk common ground: strabismus and amblyopia, not Marsden balls and balance beams.

64 Develop collaborative relationships

"Introduce yourself to faculty members at local universities or community colleges," says Joel Zaba, M.A., O.D., Virginia Beach, VA, whose specialty is learning-related vision problems. "Reach out to those who work in education, child development, and counseling. Many professors publish articles as part of their professional accreditation. Opportunities can result when two different professionals collaborate, such as an optometrist and an educator focusing on the visual screening of students in an at-risk classroom."[6]

For example, Dr. Zaba has published a series of research articles with Dr. Roger Johnson, Associate Professor of Education at Old Dominion University in Norfolk, VA. Their research relates to the social and educational consequences of undetected vision problems.

These collaborative relationships, Dr. Zaba says, can lead to lecture invitations and research projects concerning the role of vision in the learning process.

65 Refer to primary care physicians

There are many instances in which you might want to refer patients to a primary care physician or specialist. "In our practice," says Bobby Christensen, O.D., F.A.A.O., Midwest City, OK, "we check the blood pressure of patients over age 30, glaucoma patients, obese patients, and any patient with health problems that could be associated with high blood pressure. High blood pressure readings or those that are creeping up suggest the need for a referral to their primary care physicians."[7]

66 Establish a referral network

Write selected physicians in your community. Explain that you are in the process of establishing a network of primary care physicians and specialists to whom you can refer patients who are new to the area or without a physician, and request information about *their* practices.

TIP

Keep such a letter *low-key*. Don't include a brochure about your practice, article reprints, or business cards. These are self-serving and will be seen as such.

REALITY CHECK

The response to such a letter depends on a number of factors, including how swamped with patients the physician's practice is, the perceived sincerity of your letter (i.e., whether or not it appears self-serving), his or her knowledge of optometry's capabilities, and perhaps even the stationery on which it is written. In some cases, it has opened doors, prompted physicians to pick up the phone to request further information, and, down the line, resulted in reciprocal referrals.

67 Retina specialists

Low vision specialist Randall T. Jose, O.D., F.A.A.O., Houston, TX, suggests "not only contacting retina specialists, but once you have their interest, bring in lunch for the staff and spend 30 minutes with them describing the type of patients who will most benefit from low vision services."[8]

68 Co-management of vision therapy

Brenda Heinke Montecalvo, O.D., Dayton, OH, has developed a successful program for co-managing vision therapy with optometric colleagues. She recommends "once you have built a relationship, you can provide the optometrist with a co-management packet of information if he or she has not already asked for one. Include a Co-Management Mission Statement such as

> *To provide area eye care practitioners the opportunity to give their patients state-of-the-art visual therapy for learning and rehabilitation by becoming a resource for educational materials, consultation, and co-management of vision therapy.*

"Include also written assurances that the co-managed patient will return to the original eye care provider for all optical services, contact lenses and routine vision care. Co-management," she concludes, "is a real win-win proposition, for both optometrists and the patients they serve."[9]

69 Interoffice relationships

"Cultivate the relationship between your office staff and the physician's staff," says consultant Gil Weber, M.B.A., former Managed Care Director for the American Academy of Ophthalmology. "This is crucial to your successful participation as co-manager. Your office manager must meet on a regular basis with the physician's practice administrator or designate. Keep the lines of communication open, and make both practices work from the same patient care and administrative scripts. Don't make the mistake of thinking that co-management is automatic, or that an ophthalmologist will continue with it simply because you refer patients."[10]

70 Newsletters to referring physicians

A California dermatologist sends periodic newsletters to referring physicians. The first issue included the following:

> *Dear Colleague,*
> *This newsletter is being sent to you with the hope it will provide helpful information for you on the newest developments in dermatology. It's also a "thank you" for the confidence you have shown by referring patients to us.*
> *If you have any questions regarding dermatology, please don't hesitate to call. I am most happy to help you in any way I can in the management and care of your patients.*
> *Sincerely,*

Some specialists include in such newsletters a "guest columnist" from their network of referring physicians with his or her resume and a photograph. This makes the newsletter more interesting and informative. It's also a great way to cement a referral relationship.

71 Reports to teachers, pediatricians, parents, and others

"With the patient's/parent's permission, send reports to teachers, school nurse, principal, pediatrician, allergist, psychologist, physical or occupational therapist," says Anne Barber, O.D., Fullerton, CA. "Be sure also to send a copy of the report to the patient/parents. In addition to providing information about their patient/student, this also introduces many of these professionals to behavioral vision care. Even though many will not refer patients, it lays the groundwork for personal communication. And sometimes, after many reports, a pediatrician comes across a case that *does* get referred to you. Never give up communicating what you do."[11]

72 School nurses

When the AOA asked affiliated state association executive directors about referral sources, *school nurses* were ranked second after family physicians. With their important role in mind, the AOA conducted a focus group of school nurses and asked how the AOA and optometry could assist them in their duties. As a result of an overwhelming response, the AOA Communications Group School Nurse Project Team initiated a pilot project in three states: Oregon, South Dakota, and Wyoming. In each state, school nurses were sent the AOA publication entitled, *The School Nurse's Guide to Vision Screening and Ocular Emergencies*. The results were impressive: 90% of the nurses rated the materials a 1 or 2, with 1 being the most helpful and 5 being the least. In Wyoming, doctors of optometry have been asked to present education at the Nurses Association state meeting. Oregon's key person approach has facilitated new doctor of optometry/registered nurse relationships. The *School Nurse News* liked the material so well that it published the Guide in three parts.[12]

73 Primary care physicians

"Send a carefully worded, professional report to the primary care physician about every patient you schedule for an additional glaucoma workup," says Jay D. Petersma, O.D., Johnston, IA. "This tells that doctor that you treat glaucoma among other things, and it can generate referrals. Keep those letters brief," adds Dr. Petersma. "One page is enough. That physician doesn't care what the refraction was, or that the cornea was clear and the lids and lashes were free of scurf and collarettes. The issue is glaucoma."[13]

74 Co-management with ophthalmologists

"The co-management relationship starts with an assessment of clinical skills by both optometrists and ophthalmologists," says Randall N. Reichle, F.A.A.O., Houston, TX. "Neither party should assume that initials behind a name guarantee competency. You should rely on your own observations by asking ophthalmologists if they would allow you to see patients with them in their offices, observe several surgeries, and review a random selection of patient charts. The ophthalmologists can cover patients' names to protect confidentiality. Reviewing five to ten charts will give you insight into the care of any doctor. Be prepared to provide ophthalmologists the same access to your patient charts."[14]

75 Oculoplastic co-management

Oculoplastic co-management may prove to be lucrative for optometry as more types of surgeons are branching out into eyelid surgery, says Eric Schmidt, O.D., Elizabethtown, NC. "You'll get involved with not only oculoplastic surgeons but the regular plastic surgeons, some oral surgeons and maxillofacial surgeons. Most of them don't have visual field instruments, so the patients will end up paying full-fee for the surgery. You can inform those doctors that the patient may be able to get insurance to cover a portion of the surgery by having a visual field test done to prove that the blepharoplasty will improve their field of vision and hence, improve their lifestyle. This is an avenue to increase referrals to the optometrist's practice."[15]

76 Cosmetic surgeons

Are cosmetic surgeons in your area aware of tinted and opaque contact lenses? How they can enhance or change eye color? How they can improve a person's appearance? Their appearance-conscious patients are, by definition, ideal candidates.

Scott Coleman, D.D.S., F.A.G.D., Houston, TX, whose special interest is cosmetic dentistry, asked a cosmetic surgeon he knew socially if his chapter of the American Academy of Cosmetic Surgery would be interested in a talk on the subject of "How Dentistry Can

Improve a Person's Appearance." The answer was "yes." A well-received presentation led, in turn, to a network of cosmetic surgeons from whom Dr. Coleman receives frequent referrals and to whom he is able to refer patients expressing an interest in cosmetic surgery.

77 Physical therapists

Consultant Thomas D. Lecoq, Lake Forest, CA, recommends that optometrists engaged in behavioral/developmental practice start their network building with physical therapists. "Many work with head injury and stroke patients. Many of these patients recover movement quite well but report to their therapist that they are often dizzy, disoriented, see double, or see the world as 'swimming.' Such patients," he adds, "often find it impossible to go back to work or school. A growing number of articles in optometric journals address these problems yet few physical therapists have read them."

Mr. Lecoq suggests sending one of these articles with a cover letter stating, "This article deals with problems you may see in many of your patients. I thought you might find this interesting." Then include a summary of the main points of the article in one or two paragraphs. Lastly, state that because you work with patients with physical impairments, you would appreciate the opportunity to visit the therapist's office to learn more about what he or she is doing. "Don't try to convince them of your value in one session," he advises. "Take your time. Let them set the pace."[16]

78 Faulty perceptions

"What is the perception of your practice among primary care practitioners? What do they feel is the scope of your practice? We like to think our referring physicians understand what we are capable of treating, but often they do not." These questions were raised not by an optometrist, but by Marybeth Crane, a *podiatrist* in Grapevine, TX. "I had a pediatrician who sent me all of his warts and toenails," she says, "but sent calcaneal apophysitis and other 'orthopedic injuries' to the local orthopod. I sent him a referral letter on one of his patients who had a soccer injury, and this prompted a lunch discussion of childhood sports injuries. Now he sends me everything below the ankle. As a result, I increased my referrals from him by at least two patients per week just by having a 10-minute lunch conversation," she says. "Never be afraid to educate other doctors on podiatry," she adds. "You'll be surprised how misinformed they are about our profession."[17]

The problems and solutions are similar for optometry.

79 Case history is the gateway

"The questions that parents, teachers, pediatricians, occupational therapists, psychologists, speech pathologists, and reading specialists have about children's visual functioning range from basic eye health and visual acuity concerns to visual perceptual performance," says Drew J. Brooks, O.D., Brookfield, WI. "Answering them effectively helps build a referral relationship with the asking party. You'll become known as someone who knows and understands children's visual problems."[18]

What prompts these inquiries? I asked Dr. Brooks.

"This is how it works," he explained. "A parent brings his or her child to the office with some vague problems related to vision and learning that were noted in school. The case history allows me to ask all the right questions, which gives the parent the confidence that I know what to look for. Reports to teachers are then generated. The report shows the teacher I've done more than address just visual acuity issues and the need for glasses. The teacher may then think of another student who seems to have a visual perception problem, and another referral is generated. It's like fishing. One day, just the right case presents itself that allows me to do more than the last O.D. did. It might be a special needs child or a child struggling in school who already is seeing an occupational or speech therapist. My background and experience with other professionals who treat kids with learning problems allows me to ask the parent the kind of questions that reassure them that I know what is going on. The case history is the gateway.

"I offer to send a report to the therapists to explain the child's vision problem or perhaps make a phone call. The therapists are typically thrilled to get a report from someone who can answer questions they've always wondered about. In time, the word gets around. And the more questions I answer, the more I'm asked. Referrals are inevitable after that. *Communication* is the key."

80 Hard-learned lessons about networking

- The common thread of each of these network-building ideas is the importance of a *relationship*. It implies that networking is not a quick fix for an ailing practice or shortage of patients. Relationships require nurturing and a long-term outlook—more like farming than manufacturing.
- It is important to realize that networking is not an "entitlement program" in which you are eligible for referrals because you want or need them. It is not giving away business cards and asking for referrals. It is not "lunch" with a professional colleague with the expectation of referrals in exchange. As one physician expressed it, "my referrals aren't for sale."
- "If you'd like to make a serious effort at incorporating sports vision into your practice," says David O. Peed, O.D., Columbus, GA, "there's a simple word that should become part of your daily vocabulary: *Team*. And there are no 'I's in team. The sooner you see yourself as an integral part of a health care team rather than as an optometrist on the periphery of things, the sooner you'll begin to reap the benefits of adding sports vision to your growing practice."[19]
- "I feel I could go into any practice of any size in any city and convince at least one M.D. to work with me," says John McCall, O.D., Crockett, TX. "All I'd have to say is 'I have many patients with needs outside of my scope of care. As long as you respect my right to practice within my scope of care, we can work together on meeting their needs. We'll increase the draw for both of our practices.'"[20]

- "You're better off finding top-of-the-line specialists in ophthalmology (corneal, glaucoma, retinal, and cataract)—developing good rapport and referring patients to them—then, you are spreading your referrals among many ophthalmologists," says James C. Leadingham, O.D., Ashland, KY. "Everyone wins with that strategy."
- Some optometrists make these initial networking contacts, perhaps exchange information, and if it does not generate immediate referrals, they give up on the idea. "Been there, done that," they say. What they fail to recognize is that networking is an ongoing process, not a one-time event.
- "Seventy percent of my practice is M.D.-referral based," says Arthur B. Epstein, O.D., F.A.A.O., Roslyn, NY. "When we got TPAs, I was very concerned it was going to have a significant dampening effect on the practice. Fortunately, it hasn't. I think it's actually led to greater respect and greater understanding between optometry and ophthalmology, and I think this will hold true for the profession as we continue to evolve."[21]
- In the words of urologist Neil Baum, M.D., New Orleans, LA, the cultivation of physician referrals takes "patience, persistence, and prompt reporting."

81 Public speaking

Optometrists who do public speaking tend to have better practices than those who do not. They are better known, more highly regarded, and get more new patients.

How does one get started? The average optometrist has all the qualifications and ability he or she needs to become an effective public speaker. It's really just an extension of in-office patient education.

FROM THE SUCCESS FILES

"In-office seminars for educators and school nurses have played an important role in the development of my vision therapy practice," says Paul Harris, O.D., Cockeysville, MD. "To start, I had a staff member call every elementary school, both private and public, in a 10-mile radius of my office and request the name of the principal, school nurse, special education teacher, and reading instructor. Eight weeks before the program, I sent a flyer to everyone on the list. A second flyer was sent 2 weeks prior to the event. RSVP was requested, but only a handful responded."

"That first in-office seminar was almost my last one," says Dr. Harris. "A total of *four* people showed up. The seminar, however, went well. The people seemed to like the information, asked good questions, and stayed until the end and well beyond.

"The next day, two new patients were on the books as a result of the seminar. Over the next month, four more patients made appointments for vision therapy workups. This came at a critical time in the development of my practice when, to meet my growth projections, I needed one new vision therapy case every 2 weeks. This one seminar put me nearly 2 months ahead of schedule. I was hooked. For the first few years, I did six seminars a year. The following topics have always done best:

- The Relationship between Vision and Learning
- Reducing the Needs of Children with Attention Deficit Disorder/ Attention Deficit Hyperactivity Disorder
- The Remediation of Reversals
- Visualization, Visual Imagery, and Spelling
- Sports Vision

Other topics I thought would have appeal, but did not draw well, included the following:

- Myopia, Its Causes and How to Fix It
- How to Reduce Video Display Terminal (VDT) Vision Stress
- Vision and Music—How Improving Vision Can Make You a Better Musician

In-office seminars continue to be major part of my public relations efforts. Many of the sessions now have 15–25 in attendance, with one-third to one-half usually being totally new to the practice. This is an excellent source of a steady stream of new patients into the practice."

82 Speak to business and professional groups

"Educate the community on computer vision care," says Mark D. Hansen, O.D., Muscatine, IA, current President of the Iowa Optometric Association. "This should become a big part of the practice's overall computer vision effort. Look for opportunities to speak before key audiences—Parent-Teacher Associations, educators, area corporations, chambers of commerce. In many cases, employers welcome such presentations as a way of preventing potential workplace-related complaints (in this case, visual stress) and a potential opportunity to help their employees who use computers become more productive."[22]

• Ron Melton, O.D., who practices at Charlotte Eye, Ear, Nose, and Throat in Charlotte, NC, lectures to pharmacists on local and state levels in North Carolina. The topic: "Therapeutic Drug Update." "Encouraging patients to use OTC [over-the-counter] antiallergy products either actively or passively," says Dr. Melton, "may not be in their best interests because they may continue to self-medicate inappropriately. It's better to write a prescription for a drug for which we have scientific and clinical knowledge of its effectiveness. It also gives the physician, not the patient, control over drug exposure duration.[23]

"I see several of the local pharmacists as a result of this exposure," says Dr. Melton, "and they are an active source for referrals."

• "When our doctor recently spoke to a group of school psychologists," says April Nolan, assistant to behavioral optometrist Janet Kohtz, O.D., Riverside, CA, "we soon realized that the kids they were most interested in getting help for were those who lacked self-esteem. Right away, they saw the connection between visual problems, learning problems, self-esteem, and inappropriate or violent behavior in the classrooms and on the playgrounds. Already they're referring patients and we held the talk just a week ago."[24]

83 Combine public speaking with community service

Offer to conduct a short program for local service personnel (e.g., police, firefighters, school nurses, hospital emergency room staff, ambulance squad) on the subject "How to Tell if an Unconscious Victim Is Wearing Contact Lenses and How to Safely Remove Them."

REALITY CHECK

The optometrist whose only motive for public speaking is to *obtain new patients* will come across as self-serving and leave a negative impression. To avoid any misinterpretation of your motives, make little or no reference to your practice as such, your years of experience, expertise, or patients. Keep it informative and *low-key*. The idea is to establish yourself as an "authority," not as someone who is "looking for business."

84 Influential Americans

Word-of-mouth recommendations about your practice are more convincing, credible, and persuasive than any form of *self-promotion* or *paid advertising* designed to obtain new patients. That's a given.

Not all word-of-mouth recommendations, however, are equivalent. Some referral sources are *more* convincing, credible, and persuasive than others: *The Influential Americans* are one such group.

Who are they?

According to studies by the Roper Organization, a leading market research company in New York City, Influential Americans represent 10–12% of the adult population. They live up to their name as people who actively influence others. They're highly regarded and trusted; regularly asked for advice on all kinds of questions, both personal and professional; and their influence is most important for products and services that depend on word-of-mouth recommendation, like eye care, laser in situ keratomileusis surgery, and contact lenses.

Roper defines an *Influential American* as someone who has done three or more of the following in the past year: attended a public meeting, written a legislator, been an officer or committee member of a local organization, attended a political speech or rally, made a speech, written a letter to the editor, worked for a political party, worked for an activist group, written an article, and held or ran for a political office.

Influential Americans are predominantly in their 30s and 40s and married and have children. They are wealthier, better educated, hold higher-level jobs, and are more time pressured than most Americans. They put a priority on health and fitness. Of 14 exercise activities, ranging from calisthenics to swimming, 86% of Influential Americans do at least one of them on a regular basis.

This combination of education, activity, and high income gives these influential people "an insatiable thirst for knowledge and information," says Tom Miller, senior vice president of the Roper Organization. According to the report, the more information and less "hard sell" you give these influential people, the better your chances of persuading them.

TRENDSETTERS

Pioneer consumers. Trendsetters. Bellwether consumers. Leading-edge buyers. Experimenters. Early adopters. All of these terms have been used to describe Influential Americans. Why? Because this group leads the pack in accepting new products and activities. Influential Americans popularized Pilates and were using Palm Pilots long before the neighbors knew what they were. Influential Americans were also the first to fly the Concorde, buy digital cameras, and vacation in Tahiti.

The critical point is that Influential Americans are typically trendsetters, and their acceptance or rejection of a product or service can mean the difference between success and failure.

If you're involved with networking, it's a group you definitely want to reach.

WHERE TO FIND THEM

The Roper report also says that Influential Americans are social butterflies. They are avid communicators on a personal level, and enthusiastic patrons of social activities, whether they're entertaining friends at home; attending church get-togethers; going out to a nightclub; or writing, telephoning, or e-mailing a family member. They're nearly four times as likely as average Americans to attend meetings of a club or civic organization, and such activities greatly extend their sphere of influence.

Perhaps most significantly, Influential Americans carry more weight in the marketplace than their numbers and buying power would suggest. Why? Because people trust them and ask them for advice. According to the report, these people are two, three, or four times more likely than the average person to be asked for advice on a particular product or service, and are much more likely to give advice concerning such topics as health, government, politics, children, restaurants, computers, insurance, investments, cars, sports, art, and music.

Making a good impression on just one Influential American, the report says, can create *six* brand loyal customers. It's reasonable to assume their professional referrals have an equal amount of clout.

INFLUENTIAL AMERICANS TAKE ACTION

The Roper report points out that Influential Americans hold high standards for quality and performance, and take action if they're dissatisfied. They tend to complain more readily, and they stop buying a product or leave a service provider if they're disappointed. They also broadcast a negative experience to their wide network of friends and colleagues. "Influentials, a crowd easily given to action, are an unfortunate group to alienate with poor quality or poor service," the report states.

ACTION STEPS

If you're interested in increasing the numbers and clout of your referral sources, consider networking with Influential Americans in the kinds of activities in which they are actively engaged, and be sure to address their needs and priorities in your practice.[25]

Notes

1. Zwerling MH. On Finding Success in Practice. *Medical Economics*, February 19, 2001, 97.
2. Leadingham JC. How to Get More Referrals from Family Physicians. *High Performance Optometry*, March 1990, 3.
3. Epstein AB. How I Earned Hospital Privileges in New York City. *Optometric Management, Growing Your Therapeutic Practice* (supplement to *Optometric Management*), August 1998, 17S.
4. Sullins WD Jr. How Tiny Patients Made Us Better Doctors. *Review of Optometry*, July 2001, 45–46,48.
5. Brooks R. A Ruthian Approach to Diabetes. *Review of Optometry*, September 2000, 24.
6. Zaba J. Focusing on the Learning Disabled. *Optometric Management,* December 1996, 28,31,33,35.
7. Christensen B. Have You Added These Procedures? *Optometric Management,* August 1998, 8S–9S.
8. De Long S. Low Vision: How to Get Started. *Eyecare Business*, August 2000, 40,42,44.

9. Montecalvo BH. Co-Managing Vision-Therapy Patients, *Tips For Growing Your Practice*. Santa Ana, CA: Optometric Extension Program Foundation, 2000, 3–7.

10. Weber G. Blending LASIK with Traditional Vision Plans. *Optometric Management*, December 2000, 26–31.

11. Barber A. Communication: Speaking and Listening Skills. *Tips for Growing Your Practice*, Optometric Extension Program Foundation, 2000, 24–29.

12. Memo from Kenji Hamada, O.D., Chair, American Optometric Association Communications Group, August 24, 2000.

13. Petersma JD. Raise the Pressure on Glaucoma. *Optometric Management*, May 2000, 64–65,67,69.

14. Reichle RN. Exploring the Co-Management Factors You Need to Consider Before Co-Managing a Patient. *Optometric Management*, October 1998.

15. Watson D. Perimetry Can Help Detect Macular Changes, Suspected Neurologic Disease. *Primary Care Optometry News*, October 2000, 22.

16. Lecoq TD. *Developing the Dynamic Vision Therapy Practice*, edited by Willard B. Bleything, Santa Ana, CA: Optometric Extension Program Foundation, 1998.

17. Crane M. Grassroots Marketing. *Podiatry Management*, May 2001, 69–76.

18. Brooks DJ. Developing a Child and Youth Centered Practice. *Optometric Economics*, August 1993, 11,13–17.

19. Peed DO. Connecting with Other Professionals. *Optometric Management*, April 1997, 10S–11S.

20. McCall J. Succeeding in Optometric Medicine. *Optometric Management*, August 1998, 14S–17S.

21. Epstein AB. Talking TPAs, Four Conversations You Need to Hear. *Optometric Management*, March 1999, 13S.

22. Hansen MD. Nine Steps to Computer Vision Practice. *Optometry*, April 2002, 253–254.

23. Melton R. Diagnostic Challenges in Allergy Patients. *Optometric Management*, August 2001, 3–5.

24. Barber A. *Optometry's Role in Juvenile Delinquency Remediation*. Santa Ana, CA: Optometric Extension Program Foundation, 2000, 52.

25. *The Influential Americans*. The Roper Organization, 1992.

5

Getting to "Yes"

Nothing happens in optometry until the patient says "yes." And *patient education* holds the key to achieving that. The better educated patients are, the more they'll comply with home care instructions, and the more they'll say "yes" to periodic comprehensive exams, refractive surgery, vision therapy, recalls, contact lenses, prescription lenses for occupational and avocational purposes, premium lens options, and on and on.

"Take the time to teach," say Joseph T. Barr, O.D., M.S., F.A.A.O., and Timothy B. Edrington, O.D., M.S., Editor and Contributing Editor, respectively, of *Contact Lens Spectrum*. "With contact lens consumerism at an all-time high (or low, depending on your perspective), it is critical for you and your staff to expend a greater effort in educating your patients about eye care and eyewear options. If you don't, your competition will."[1]

REALITY CHECK

In the first study of its kind, nearly 500 patients of 74 internists were asked to list, in order of importance, nine major components of medical care. Patients listed "communication of information" second in importance, right after medical skill. Where did that item rank in doctors' opinions? *Sixth* on the list.

"This certainly indicates that doctors underestimate patients' desire for more information," says the author of the study, Christine Laine, M.D., M.P.H., assistant professor of medicine at Jefferson Medical College, Philadelphia, PA.[2]

85 Inform before you perform

Many patients worry and sometimes agonize about whether they've given the right answers during subjective testing.

Mark R. Sukoenig, O.D., Syracuse, NY, recommends explaining to patients *why* you are doing *what* you are doing. For example

"You can't make a mistake reading the eye chart during an eye exam. What I'm asking you to do is to tell me what the letters look like to you. Whatever you tell me is correct."

Here's another: "If I ask you, 'which is better, one or two?' and you're not sure, that's OK. That's exactly the answer I'm looking for."

"Sometimes," he continues, "it'll be easy for you to tell which is better. I'm trying to find the point at which it's hard to tell the difference."[3]

Another example of the need to "inform before you perform" involves computer vision syndrome (CVS).

"To best serve your patients who have CVS," says Peter G. Shaw-McMinn, O.D., co-author of *The Care and Management of the Computer Syndrome Patient* (Butterworth–Heinemann, 2002), "you must educate them before you examine them, and continue to do so throughout the visit. The earlier you begin educating your patients about CVS, the more likely they will be to follow your recommendations."[4]

"When referring a patient for refractive surgery," say Bruce A. Krawiecki, O.D., and Geoffrey C. Calaway, O.D., Houston, TX, "take control of his care. Make sure your patient understands that you will provide all pre- and postoperative care, including prescribing medications. After you've discussed the surgery thoroughly with your patient, call the surgeon's office to schedule the appointment. Be confident in your referral. Don't leave anything to chance, particularly with regards to when the patient will return to you for follow-up."[5]

86 Show understanding

"As any long-time contact lens practitioner knows," says Janice M. Jurkis, O.D., M.B.A., F.A.A.O., Chicago, IL, and Carol A. Schwartz,

O.D., M.B.A., F.A.A.O., Vista, CA, "one of the biggest obstacles to contact lenses (and the hardest to get the patient to admit to) is *fear*, the most common form of which is touching the eye."[6]

One technique for dealing with such concerns is called the Feel-Felt-Found formula.

Mrs./Mr. Smith, I know how you *feel*. Many patients have *felt* exactly the same way. But, after a little practice, they *found* that this was far simpler and easier to do than was initially thought. You will too.

The "Feel-Felt-Found" formula is just a track to run on and should, of course, be adapted to the situation. It is simply intended to acknowledge patients' concerns and to let them know their feelings are perfectly normal and reasonable under the circumstances and that other people have felt exactly the same way. What this does is to make patients less self-conscious about their fears. It also spares them the added embarrassment of thinking they're acting foolishly and everyone will think less of them.

87 The single most important factor in patient acceptance

Patients do not accept your recommendations for periodic comprehensive eye examinations, refractive surgery, and vision therapy because they understand the fine points of what's involved. They do so because, in a word, they *trust* you.

POWER OF TRUST

Morton Salt, the world's leading producer of salt, conducted focus groups to learn why its customers were willing to pay a little more for its salt, even though it is identical to all other salt. The company admitted to the participants that its salt was *identical* to that of its competitors and even that it supplied salt to others who sold it for a lower price.

The group members responded they would *still* buy Morton's salt at the higher price because they *trusted* the company more than others to provide a fair measure and a clean, uncontaminated product.[7] *Trust*, in this case, is what has given Morton Salt its competitive advantage.

Is this applicable in optometry? You bet!

ACTION STEPS

How do you develop a patient's trust? It's a question I've asked countless health care practitioners. The reply I like best was from Mitchell T. Cantor, D.M.D., M.S.D., a periodontist in Southampton, Long Island, NY, who told me, "Be very slow to get into the patient's mouth. First, get into the patient's *heart*; then, the patient's *head*; and *then*, into the patient's mouth."

The concept is as applicable to optometry as it is to periodontics.

- Go s-l-o-w-l-y. I have always advocated prescribing for a patient's vocational and avocational vision needs. But trying to do it *all*, especially on a patient's *first* visit, may be construed as "high pressure" and may undermine trust.
- Be low-key. Frederic A. Munz, O.D., Wake Forest, NC, says, "I tell patients: 'It's my job to present you with the best vision, health, and comfort options we have. It's your job to select which options are meaningful to you.'"[8]
- Keep your promises. "If you say that the glasses will be ready on Tuesday," says Dr. Munz, "and they're not here on Tuesday, you've ruined your credibility."[8]
- "Trust emerges when a patient feels cared about as a person, when the patient believes you are sensitive and caring, and when the patient senses you are trying to understand his or her feelings," says Charles L. Millone, D.D.S.[9]
- "There is no faster way to build a foundation of trust," says consultant Susan Keane Baker, "than to be absolutely fanatical about patient confidentiality. Letting a patient know you are committed to patient confidentiality will cement your relationship faster than almost anything else you can do."[10]
- Requiring staff members to sign confidentiality agreements on an annual basis is a good way to maintain awareness of the importance of protecting patients' privacy.
- Be willing to refer cases beyond your scope of practice and comfort zone to another practitioner better qualified to deal with the case.

FROM THE SUCCESS FILES

Dr. Lyle R. Jackson, a veterinarian in Salt Lake City, UT, expressed it well when he told me, "No veterinarian can have all the skills and equipment to do everything. If we perform a procedure, it's because we can do it as well or better than any veterinarian in the Salt Lake City area. If not, we refer the client and say, "For this procedure, there's another doctor who can do it better. That's not in our best interest, but it's in yours. And that's what matters most."

Some practitioners fear that patients will think less of them if they refer a difficult case to a more qualified colleague. Just the contrary happens: Surveys show that patients admire and appreciate doctors who willingly refer special procedures and forgo revenue in the process.

By the same token, patients don't expect a doctor of optometry to be good at everything. When you admit your limitations, you *gain* rather than lose stature in your patients' eyes. Your honesty makes you more human and credible. And, as Dr. Jackson also noted, it reduces your malpractice risks.

---

88 Present pros *and* cons

Patients tend to be impressed with, and have more trust in, optometrists who explain the *pros* and *cons* of such recommendations as progressive addition lenses; disposable contacts; and, in the case of laser-assisted in situ keratomileusis (LASIK) surgery, the risks. It imbues their recommendations with a sense of balance. Makes them more believable.

FROM THE SUCCESS FILES

Investing his own time and money and refusing to accept any advertising, Brian Chou, O.D., Los Angeles, CA, created his own watch-dog Web site about the benefits and drawbacks of laser vision correction (http://www.refractivesource.com). The purpose? To give potential patients an impartial look at the pros and cons of refractive surgery.

The site includes an essay on presbyopia and refractive surgery, lists requirements for the procedure, and explains why realistic expectations are vital when deciding whether to go through with LASIK. The main goal of Refractive Source is to emphasize that although LASIK and other refractive surgical procedures offer excellent alternatives to glasses or contact lenses, they are still effective only for carefully selected patients with specific vision needs.

"The results can be life-changing," cautions Dr. Chou, "and it is therefore important to understand what you're getting into and what to expect before having it done."[11]

Financier J. P. Morgan best summed up the importance of trust: "The client's belief in the integrity of our advice is our most valuable possession."

89 Use visual aids

University studies show that people retain only 11% of what they hear versus 83% of what they see. Obviously, patient education, to be *effective*, needs a strong visual component.

FROM THE SUCCESS FILES

- "Corneal topography has been a good tool for us," says David W. Hansen, O.D., Des Moines, IA. "The topographer lets you see dry eye conditions which you can show patients on the corneal maps."[12]
- "Technicians at the practice of R. Whitman Lord, O.D., with five locations in Georgia, use retinal digital photography on all patients older than age 16 years. Those images are displayed on monitors throughout the practice, so when a patient enters an examination room, he can see an image of his retina. That leads to a discussion of his retinal health," says Dr. Lord, "and patients like the high-tech aspect of seeing their retinal pictures on a computer screen."[12]
- When discussing the importance of yearly dilated exams to patients with diabetes, Dan Bintz, O.D., Elk City, OK, simply hits a couple of keys on his computer keyboard and brings up a fundus photo showing a patient with diabetic retinopathy. He then explains this disease is often preventable with good control and is

treatable when problems are found early. If ignored, this disease can lead to blindness.

- A video slit-lamp is another highly convincing visual aid. "A lot of times," says Donald Higgins, O.D., Plainsville, CT, "patients don't realize how bad their contact lenses are, whether it's a scratch on a gas permeable lens or jelly bumps on a soft lens. Once patients are shown their damaged or deposit-laden lenses on the monitor," he says, "I have no problem convincing them it's time for new lenses." [13]

- Model of the eye: "This is a must for explaining the parts of the eye and how they all fit together," says Larry E. Harris, O.D., Topeka, KS. "For instance, if a patient is seeing floaters, I can show the posterior chamber and explain why the floaters are occurring. I even use it to explain a fundus photo. You'd be surprised," he adds, "how many patients don't understand which part of the eye is being photographed." [14]

- Two excellent take-home visual aids are also available from the American Optometric Association. One is a full-color reproduction of the fundus of the human eye (item G-10); the other, a schematic section of the human eye (item G-11). Both forms have all parts labeled and definitions printed on the reverse side. These forms, which you can personalize by drawing arrows, for example, help patients better understand and remember your explanations. Patients often show them to family members and, in many cases, they end up as "show and tell" in their children's schoolroom classes.

RECOMMENDED RESOURCE

Take-apart anatomical models of the eye and forms G-10 and G-11 are available from the Order Department of the American Optometric Association, 243 North Lindberg Blvd., St. Louis, MO 63141-7881, (800) 365-2219.

REALITY CHECK

With the pressure we're under today to do more exams and do them faster, some optometrists say that patient education is just too time consuming.

Perception or reality?

I've used an egg timer at seminars to dramatize just how long three minutes can be. It is considerably longer than most people realize and more than enough time to upgrade a patient's "optometric IQ."

90 Keeping contact lens patients compliant

One way to keep patients from dropping out is to make sure they care for their lenses properly and follow the recommended wearing schedules. Stressing the latter is important, especially when it comes to disposable and frequent replacement lenses.

FROM THE SUCCESS FILES

- Thomas R. Lentz, O.D., Wichita, KS, has two sets of photographs he shows patients. The first is a healthy eye; the second set demonstrates what can happen if the patient doesn't follow his prescribed wearing schedule. "Patients can be overwhelmed by the amount of instructions and verbal information we give them," he says, "but visualization is something they usually remember."[12]
- Timothy B. Edrington, O.D., M.S., chief of contact lens services at Southern California College of Optometry, and Joseph T. Barr, O.D., M.S., F.A.A.O., assistant dean of Clinical Affairs at the Ohio State University College of Optometry, have this recommendation: "At the dispensing visit, discuss the appropriate wearing-time schedule, problematic signs and symptoms and how patients should respond, lens application and removal, proper care of the lenses and lens case (don't simply refer the patient to the package insert or the instructions on the box), the lens replacement schedule, and the rationale for why each one of these instructions is in the patient's best interest."[1]
- Larry K. Wan, O.D., Campbell, CA, recommends that when contact lens patients pay their bills, it is important for staff members to reinforce proper contact lens care and storage, proper wearing schedule, proper replacement schedule, and emergency phone numbers.[15]

91 Monitor patients' understanding

Ask patients to repeat your instructions in their own words. Consultant Jacob Weisberg calls this *reverse paraphrasing* and says it is far more effective than repeating the same points over and over. "Reverse paraphrasing lets you know how well the patient understands your instructions," Mr. Weisberg says. "If you just *tell* patients and don't get any inkling of what they've understood, then the chances of compliance are reduced."[16]

In the management of glaucoma, says Murray Fingeret, O.D., Optometry Section, St. Albans Veterans Administration, St. Albans, NY, "questions can be used to sample whether the patient is adhering to the regimen." For example

"Did you get the prescription filled?
Show me how you take this medication.
Do you stop taking the medication when your eyes feel better?
Do you stop taking the medication if you experience discomfort?
When do you take the medication?
Do you know how long you need to take the medication?
Do you know why you are taking the medication?"

"While certain portions of the exam can be delegated," says Dr. Fingeret, "the interview, as well as the closing, can only be done by the optometrist taking care of the patient. It is during this time that patients get to understand their condition and their role in management."[17]

"Have glaucoma patients show you how they use the drops," suggests Jay Petersma, O.D., Des Moines, IA. "I find the single most important aspect of compliance and effectiveness of medication is proper technique of applying eye drops."[18]

REALITY CHECK

"An astounding number of patients," says Sherrie Kaplan, co-director of the Primary Care Outcomes Research Institute, Boston, MA, "anywhere from 30% to 60% by various researchers' counts, do not take medications as their doctors prescribe. For some chronic diseases in which good self-care and following physicians' instructions count most, the numbers on patient adherence are utterly dismal. Diabetes? Somewhere between 40–50% of patients neglect to follow the suggested drug regimen. Hypertension? Forty percent fail to comply. Arthritis? Up to 70% of patients don't follow doctors' orders when it comes to medication."[19]

"I was flabbergasted to learn that a third of my patients never fill the prescriptions I give them," says Stuart Thomas, O.D., Athens, GA, a participant in the Alcon/National Data Corporation (NDC Health) Study.[20]

92 Use positive reinforcement

B. F. Skinner is the psychologist generally credited with discovering the power of positive reinforcement, a behavior modification technique that can greatly improve patient compliance.

In some of his early experiments, Skinner found that any random act of a pigeon would be repeated if it was immediately reinforced with value (a kernel of corn). Thus, if he wanted a pigeon to peck a disc the size of a quarter, he would reinforce the pigeon with corn if the pigeon just happened to peck near the disc. If it pecked the disc itself, it would get several kernels. After a short time, the pigeon would peck the disc and keep on pecking it any number of times.

Skinner discovered that people, too, would repeat behavior, which was immediately reinforced with "value." They didn't even have to know they were being reinforced. The "value" could be psychological reinforcement such as praise, recognition, or appreciation.

Other psychologists have used such reinforcers as a smile, a head nod, and the words "fine," "good," and even a "hmmm" to get subjects to be more communicative, express more personal opinions, and ask more questions, all without the subject realizing what was happening.

There are countless ways for you and your staff to harness the power of positive reinforcement to encourage patients to repeat desirable behavior. For example, tell them the following:

"You're always so punctual for your appointments. We really appreciate that."

"It's great that you are coming in every year to be checked. I wish all of our diabetic patients were as conscientious about this as you are."

To a patient during the exam itself: "You're doing just fine—making this easier—and helping me."

The words you use are less important than the fact that you're acknowledging someone's efforts in a way that has motivational value.

PRINCIPLE INVOLVED

Behavior that is reinforced tends to be repeated. Behavior that is ignored tends to be extinguished.

REALITY CHECK

Patients occasionally slip, going longer than a year without an exam, being late for appointments, and squirming in the chair. Applaud their successes rather than criticize their failures.

---

93 Be willing to answer questions

Today's patients are taking an increasingly active role in their health by asking questions about their condition. Doctors who do not take the time to adequately answer such questions or, worse, who appear to *resent* them, often *lose* patients. Unfortunately, the loss doesn't stop there as the story of the doctor's indifference or arrogance is repeated over and over.

Some of the questions originate on Web sites such as that of the National Eye Institute (http://www.nei.nih.gov/publications/tips.htm), where, for example, there is a page entitled: "Tips for Talking to Your Doctor." It includes a page of questions for patients to ask about their condition, such as the following:

- *Diagnosis* (e.g., What caused my condition? Can it be treated?)
- *Treatment* (e.g., What are the risks and side effects? Are other treatments available?)
- *Tests* (e.g., What do you expect to find out from these tests?)

It is then followed by a section entitled "Understanding Your Doctor's Responses Is Essential to Good Communication," which includes these additional tips:

- If you don't understand your doctor's responses, ask questions until you do understand.
- Take notes, or get a friend or family member to take notes for you. Or, bring a tape recorder to assist in your recollection of the discussion.
- Ask your doctor to write down his or her instructions to you.
- Ask your doctor for printed material about your condition.
- If you still have trouble understanding your doctor's answers, ask where you can go for more information.

FROM THE SUCCESS FILES

"Instead of being threatened by a patient who brings me information from the Internet," says gynecologist Neeta Ambe-Crain, M.D., Thousand Oaks, CA, "I try to compliment her for taking such a proactive interest in her health."[21]

REALITY CHECK

One-half of America's 100 million households changed, added, or selected a physician in the past 2 years, according to a recent study by VHA Inc., an Orlando, FL–based network of community-owned hospitals.

Contrary to popular assumptions, health plans are not the top reason for this record change, the study concludes. According to VHA's findings, 52% of health care consumers say *poor communication* is the main reason they are unhappy with their present physician. Another 25% said they were not satisfied with the quality of care they received.

According to the research, 71% of health care consumers say they were given no health information during their last physician visit, yet 85% of those who did receive information found it extremely helpful. The study also found that of all the ways to obtain health information, getting information from their personal physician is most consumers' first choice.[22]

"Patients like to be involved," says Sherrie Kaplan, co-director of the Primary Care Outcomes Research Institute in Boston, MA. "Not only that," she adds, "when a physician welcomes their taking part, patients perceive this as evidence the doctor cares about them."

"Patients who ask questions, elicit treatment options, express opinions, and state preferences about treatment during office visits with physicians, have measurably better health outcomes than patients who do not," Kaplan wrote in the *Annals of Internal Medicine*. "No amount of technically excellent care will produce optimal outcomes if patients are not actively engaged in managing diseases, particularly chronic disease."[19]

94 Beware of overkill

Patient education is unquestionably the key to helping patients better understand their conditions and how best to deal with them. What you want to avoid is *overkill*, which occurs when optometrists get carried away with patient education and tell patients *more* than they want to hear or need to know.

Why do some doctors of optometry go overboard on patient education? Among the reasons are the following:

- They overestimate patients' interest in getting a detailed explanation of their condition.
- Some believe the more they explain and the more persuasive they are, the better the chances of patients saying "yes" to their recommendations.
- Others fail to notice a patient's blank stare while they are talking or other signs the patient has lost interest in what they're saying.

In short, the trap into which these well-meaning but overly talkative optometrists fall is thinking more about what they want to *say* than what the patient wants to *hear*.

If you think you may at times be guilty of "over-explaining," here's a strategy that may help. After a minute or two of nonstop talking about the etiology of dry eye, the benefits of multifocal contact lenses, or whatever the subject, *stop talking* and ask the patient: "Is this interesting?"

If the patient says, "yes," keep going. Even better, if the patient says "Yes, and you're first doctor who ever explained this to me," give yourself a pat on the back and keep talking—you've hit a home run.

If the patient replies to your question with only a shrug and a look of little interest in hearing more about the subject, however, cut your explanation short. You'll save time, prevent overkill, and have a happier patient.

"Most patients want some understanding of their condition," says Donna Higgins, O.D., Prairie du Chien, WI, "but a long, overly detailed explanation will make them 'tune out' and stop listening."[23]

95   A well-designed, informative, user-friendly Web site

"Perhaps the most important reason to have a Web site," says Gary Gerber, O.D., Hawthorne, NJ, "is that in today's high-tech information age, your patients expect it."[24]

"The effectiveness of the Web stems from its seamless integration into the daily activities and management of the practice," says Rochelle Mozlin, O.D., State University of New York College of Optometry, New York, NY. "When patients are scheduled for evaluations, they are referred to the Web site to download and complete a case history form. When patients call to ask for directions to the office, they are again directed to the Web site. After the diagnostic evaluation, they are referred to the library of vision conditions. When they complete their vision therapy program, a success story [see Chapter 8] is generated and posted on the Web site with a photograph. Each encounter with the Web site is creating a better-educated patient or parent with an orientation toward a successful outcome."[25]

RECOMMENDATION

"There are many ways to create an office Web site," says Gary Osias, O.D., San Lorenzo, CA, "but I only recommend one. Seek out the help of a professional designer and pay to have a Web site that impresses Internet surfers. Homegrown Web sites appear obviously amateur to professional computer users, and when professional computer users search the Web, they base their first impression of a business by the quality of its Web site."[26]

96 Image gap

When asked to guess the number of postgraduate courses their optometrists have taken in the last 6 months, most patients with whom I've talked have no idea. Such perceptions are disappointing but not surprising, given that most patients are never told about such courses. I call this an *image gap*.

Knowing that you and your staff attend postgraduate courses boosts patients' confidence and increases their loyalty. Do not lose these important benefits by making a secret of the continuing education that you, your associates, and staff members take.

ACTION STEP

An easy, low-cost way to inform patients is to post a notice on your Web site, a bulletin board in your reception area, or a cardboard easel at the front counter. Suggested wording is as follows:

> We will be away from the office from time to time in the coming year to attend postgraduate courses. Among them. . .(Here, list the dates, the individuals attending, the titles of the courses, and short, non-technical descriptions of the course content).

Posting such a notice has several benefits:

- Makes patients aware of your comprehensive, full scope of practice and your commitment to continuing education.
- Alerts patients to your special interests and expertise (e.g., optic nerve disease, vision therapy, low vision, CVS, infant eye and vision assessment).
- May prompt inquiries about services that patients don't realize are within the scope of your practice (e.g., glaucoma management, headaches, reading difficulties, sports vision, co-management of refractive surgery).
- Explains your, your associates', and your staff's extended absences from the office in a positive way (as opposed to having patients think you are taking numerous vacation days).

- Differentiates your practice from others.

Of course, not everyone reads such a notice or necessarily grasps its significance. But more than you might guess will read it, and be interested and impressed. If nothing else, it helps your practice avoid the image gap.

97 Hard-learned lessons about patient education

- Patient education is the responsibility of every optometric team member, and every position in the practice affords the opportunity to educate.
- "Female patients ages 35–50 [years]," says Jay D. Petersma, O.D., Johnston, IA, "are a wonderful audience for just about any type of eye care education because they're commonly the health care decision-makers in the family. Also, they're often not only looking out for their own family, but are arranging health care for their parents or in-laws as well."[27]
- Telling isn't *teaching*. Listening isn't *learning*. Studies show that 1 hour after we have been exposed to new information, 56% has been forgotten. A day later, another 10% slips away.
- *Spaced repetitions* help patients remember what you tell them.
- Personalize take-home literature by using a fiber pen to circle key paragraphs or underline important points as you discuss them with patients. It increases the odds of the material being read and remembered.
- Asking patients: "Do you understand?" is one way of monitoring patient comprehension. That question, however, puts the onus on *them* to understand what may have been an overly technical or rushed explanation. Rather than look foolish, some patients *say* they understand when, in fact, they don't.
- Ask instead, "Does the way I am explaining this make sense? This phrasing puts the onus on *you* to clearly explain everything. It is also makes it easier for patients to admit they do not understand.

- If a patient asks you to clarify something you believe you have already explained, don't show exasperation, such as by taking a deep breath, audibly sighing, or talking down to the patient.

Notes

1. Edrington TB, Barr JT. Take the Time to Teach. *Contact Lens Spectrum*, July 2001, 50.
2. Laine C, Davidoff F, Lewis CE, et al. Important Elements of Outpatient Care: A Comparison of Patients' and Physicians' Opinions. *Annals of Internal Medicine*, October 1996, 640–645.
3. Sukoenig MR. What You Really Mean. *Optometric Management*, June 2001, 18.
4. Shaw-McMinn PG. CVS: The Practical and the Clinical. *Review of Optometry*, August 2001, 78–84,86–87.
5. Krawiecki BA, Calaway GC. Using Co-Management Opportunities to Build Your Practice. *Optometric Management*, November 2001, 18–19.
6. Jurkis JM, Schwartz CA. The Top Reasons Why Your Patients Don't Wear Contact Lenses. *Optometric Management*, November 2000, 67,73–75.
7. Mullen JX. Brand Power. *Bottom Line/Business*, October 1996, 15.
8. Munz FA. Strategies for Better Patient Retention. *Optometric Management*, September 2000, 3S–8S.
9. George JM, Millone CL. *Stress Management for the Dental Team.* Philadelphia: Lea & Febiger, 1986.
10. Baker SK. *Managing Patient Expectation: The Art of Finding and Keeping Loyal Patients.* San Francisco: Jossey-Bass Publishers, 1998.
11. DeAngelis T. One Doctor's Crusade to Demystify Refractive Surgery. *CONNeCTED* (supplement to *Review of Optometry*), November 2000, 10–11.
12. Keeping Your Contact Lens Patients Compliant. Healthy Patients, Healthy Practices. Supplement to *Optometric Management*, July 2001, 12S–14S.
13. Murphy R. Video Technology in the Exam Room. *Review of Optometry*, August 1993, 65.
14. Harris LE. Double Your Patient-Persuasion Power. *Optometric Management*, July 1993, 31–33.
15. Wan LK. The Annual Dispensing Advantage. *Optometric Management*, June 2001, 38–40.
16. Weiss CG. Your Patient Thought You Said What? *Medical Economics*, February 7, 2000, 249–252.

17. Fingeret M. Patient Communication—The Hidden Procedure in the Management of Glaucoma. *Optometry*, May 2001, 279.
18. Epstein AB. The Compliance Conundrum. *Review of Optometry*, July 2001, 66–74.
19. Dahl R. How to Get Through to Your Patients. *Hippocrates*, April 1997, 38–44.
20. Goodwin J. Do You Count? *Optometric Management*, April 2001, 29–30,34,36–37,101.
21. Ambe-Crain N. On Listening. *Medical Economics*, April 23, 2001, 103.
22. *Practice Marketing and Management*, June 1999, 84.
23. Higgins D. Encouraging Patients to Understand the Rationale for Routine Examination. *Optometric Management*, March 2001, 89–92.
24. Gerber G. Spin a Smaller Web. *Review of Optometry*, June 2001, 35.
25. Mozlin R. *Web VT*. Volume 11, Number 5, 2000, 115–121.
26. Osias G. You Have the Cure, So Let Patients Know It. http://www.sightstreet.com, April 18, 2001.
27. Petersma JD. Raise the Pressure on Glaucoma. *Optometric Management*, May 2000, 64–65,67,69.

6

Patient Expectations, Satisfaction, and Loyalty

"You already know that the customer is always right, right?" asks writer Lucy McCauley. "But these days—given the speed and interactivity of the Internet, the explosion of customer choice, the emergence of new competitive pressures, and the constant expansion of customers' expectations for service—just giving customers what they want isn't enough. You also have to anticipate needs, solve problems before they start, provide service that wows, and offer responses to mistakes that more than make up for the original error."[1]

This excerpt, from an article in *Fast Company*, targets the business community. It is, however, also dead-on for optometry.

Let us start at the beginning.

98 Moments of truth

Jan Carlson, President and CEO of Scandinavian Airline Systems (SAS), is credited with popularizing the term: *moment of truth*. Taken from the lexicon of bull fighting, it refers to any episode in which a passenger (or prospective passenger) comes into contact with an SAS employee. For example, moments of truth include the points at which a passenger makes a reservation, checks into the airport, boards the plane, retrieves luggage, or makes contact with an SAS employee during the flight.

As Carlson explains, "Nothing is more fragile than the fleeting contact between a customer in the marketplace and an employee on the front lines. When you establish contact, that's when you establish SAS."

"SAS has 10 million passengers a year," says Carlson. "The average passenger comes in contact with five SAS employees. Therefore, SAS is the product of the 10 million times 5 or 50 million 'moments of truth' per year—50 million unique, never-to-be-repeated opportunities to distinguish ourselves, in a memorable fashion, from each and every one of our competitors."[2]

There are countless moments of truth that occur when patients visit an optometric office that in the same way shape their image of a practice, starting with the first phone call. How many rings does it take for your phone to be answered? Is the caller given a long menu of recorded options, put on hold, and then required to listen to recorded messages before finally reaching a "live" person? Is that live person friendly and helpful or brusque and impatient? Is the caller (who may have been in your office countless times) recognized by name or asked, "Are you a patient here?" Are patients with "emergencies" given immediate advice and/or instructions or put on hold?

And this is just a phone call.

How about those moments when a patient does any of the following:

- Logs onto your Web site
- Arrives at your building
- Enters your office, perhaps accompanied by a child
- Is handed off to the technician for pretesting
- Is first greeted by the doctor
- Is examined by the doctor
- Is given an explanation of the doctor's findings and recommendations
- Is handed off to the contact lens technician or optician in the dispensary
- Pays for services at the front desk
- Departs the practice
- Returns for delivery of eyewear
- Possibly complains at the front desk

In each case, a patient's lasting impression of your practice is determined by how competent, concerned, accommodating, trustworthy, and professional you and your staff members are—not just on the first visit, but *every time* a patient calls or visits your practice.

ACTION STEP

Schedule a staff meeting to decide what impression you would most like to make on new patients. What is it that you would like them to think or say to others about their first to visit your office? There is no "correct" answer as such: It could be any one of countless things discussed in this book. If, however, you can reach a consensus on what it should be ideally, you are well on your way to making it happen.

99 Expectations gap

Our studies indicate that in the typical practice, 75% of referrals are made by only 15–20% of patients. Why so few? The answer lies in what I call the *expectations gap*, or the disparity between a patient's *expectations* about a visit to an optometric office and his or her *perception* of the experience itself.

REALITY CHECK

Yankelovich Partners Inc., one of the premier market research firms in the United States, specializes in studying consumer behavior and attitudes, often the best predictor of future marketplace behavior. Their signature product, *Monitor*, is an ongoing survey of 2,500 consumers, 16 years and older, from all parts of the country.

A recent survey concluded, "Consumers are unwilling to compromise on their high expectations. Because there are so many options, consumers do not feel compelled to "award" their business to establishments that fail to treat them with the level of customer service they have come to expect."[3]

Consumers were asked whether or not they agreed with the following statements:

- "I feel the prices I pay now for goods and services entitle me to the highest level of customer service" (*84% agreed*).
- "Most of the time, the service people that I deal with for the products and services that I buy don't care about me or my needs" (*62% agreed*).

"Companies that do express care in customer service," the report went on to say, "are not only winning business, they are raising the bar for the rest of the marketplace."

100 Degrees of patient satisfaction

It is an oversimplification to be sure, but for discussion purposes, let us divide the patients in a typical practice into three groups.

The first group is those patients who are *disappointed* by the experience of a visit to an optometric office because their expectations for quality of care, service, office environment, a friendly staff, wide selection of eyewear, and the like, were *not met*. These are *dissatisfied* patients who, depending on the severity of their complaints, may take several courses of action.

Mildly dissatisfied patients usually say nothing at the time. Most tolerate minor inconveniences, but less so if they occur on a repeated basis.

Patients with *greater* dissatisfaction speak up, in many cases repeating the story of what went wrong to their friends, acquaintances, and perhaps co-workers. Such negative word-of-mouth can seriously damage your reputation and referrals. If such patients were referred by a physician, pharmacist, or other professional, then bad reports can possibly *end* that referral relationship.

REALITY CHECK

Studies conducted by the Technical Assistance Research Programs (TARP), Washington, DC, indicate that unhappy patients tell, on average, 10–12 others about their experience. Thirteen percent of people who have had a bad experience tell 20 or more about it, often embellishing the details to make a better story.

Truly *angry* patients leave the practice, possibly notify their managed-care plan administrator, and, in the worst-case scenario, sue for malpractice.

Richard Boone, a McLean, VA, attorney who defends doctors in malpractice cases, tells me that the common denominator in every lawsuit with which he's been involved has been "failed expectations."

The second group is those patients whose expectations were *essentially met*. "The doctor was OK." "The staff was OK." "The office was OK." "The service was OK." These are *satisfied* patients.

REALITY CHECK

Many patients use the word "satisfaction" (or "OK") not so much to express positive feelings, but rather to communicate the absence of negative feelings. It often turns out to be a "neutral" feeling, which means they may or may not talk about their experience; may or may not refer anyone; may or may not even *stay* in the practice.

The third group of patients consists of those whose expectations for quality of care, service, office environment, frame selection, and so on, are *more than met*—they are *exceeded*. When asked about their experience, these patients talk in glowing terms about the "most thorough exam I've ever had," "the friendliness of the staff," "the wonderful service," and on and on. Their experience was more than "OK." They are more than satisfied. More than just "happy." These are *enthusiastic* patients, the ones who make *referrals*, who convince other family members to come to you, who *thank* the friend or physician or whoever referred them, *and* who pay their bills cheerfully and promptly. Even more important, these patients are intensely *loyal*. They will stick with you, whether or not you are a provider on their managed-care plan, have higher fees, or keep them waiting.

REALITY CHECK

In the *typical* practice, these enthusiastic patients represent the 15–20% of patients who account for 75% of referrals.

High-performance optometric practices, on the other hand, have a higher-than-average number of enthusiastic, loyal patients and, in turn, a higher-than-average number of referrals. The reason is simple: patients' expectations are greatly exceeded—not just once in a while, but on every visit.

101 Civility factor

For the annual *Yankelovich Monitor* report on values, beliefs, and lifestyles, 2,500 adult consumers are interviewed in their homes for 2 hours. They are asked hundreds of questions about their attitudes and behaviors on a wide variety of topics. Among them are "What is most important to you regarding customer service—that is, the way you are treated by business or its employees when purchasing products or services?"

The results in descending order are as follows:

Courtesy	25%
Knowledgeable	21%
Friendliness	13%
Listens to you	13%
Efficiency	10%
Thoroughness	8%
Promptness	5%
Availability	5%

What's interesting about these findings is that *efficiency*, often the focus of optometrists' efforts to improve the profitability of their practices, is significantly less important to consumers than courtesy, friendliness, and simply listening to them.

Britt Beemer, author of *Predatory Marketing* (Doubleday Bantam, 1998) is not surprised by these statistics. "Efficiency is not a replacement for customer service," he says. "It's only a small part of building relationships with customers. This blind focus on efficiency perfectly describes the breach between what customers want and what companies think they want."[4]

"The overriding message of these findings," says Barbara Kaplan, a partner at Yanklelovich Partners, Inc., "is that people want to be treated with *civility*. If they're not, they can and will go elsewhere."

The *civility factor*, as I call it, should be an important consideration when deciding whom to hire and what the priorities of your practice will be.

HARD-LEARNED LESSON

"One of the lessons to be learned about service," say consultants Karl Albrecht and Lawrence J. Bradford, Ph.D., "is that the longer a business has been in existence, the more likely it is that it has lost sight of what is important to customers."[5]

102 Learn new patients' expectations

To achieve the highest level of patient satisfaction, it is essential to know what new patients expect on a visit to your office, and what they would like to happen (or *not happen*, if they have been previously disappointed by another office). There is, however, no universal answer. No two patients have the same expectations, the same likes and dislikes, or have them in the same order of importance.

New patients often volunteer the reason they left their previous eye care practitioner; others remain closed-mouthed about it. The problem when you don't know the reason is that it leaves you and your staff in the dark as to what, if anything, went wrong and how you might prevent it from happening in your office.

Suppose the reason the patient left was because the optometrist was always late for appointments, the optician was high-pressure, or the receptionist was rude. These would alert you and your staff to specific behaviors to avoid at all possible costs. Wouldn't it be shortsighted not to know?

ACTION STEPS

Consider asking new patients during the get-acquainted portion of the first visit, the following question: "If you don't mind my asking, could you please tell me the reason you left your previous eye doctor? If there were problems of any kind, I want to make sure they don't happen here."

By telling patients your reason for asking, they're more likely to open up and tell you their true feelings. And of course, there will be patients who truly liked their previous eye care practitioner and *regretted* having to leave. If appropriate, inquire as to the reasons for their affection and loyalty so you can follow suit.

103 Manage patients' expectations

Patients often have unrealistic expectations. They can be about managed care, refractive surgery, contact lenses, or a host of other things.

Take managed care, for example. Some patients have the mistaken belief that everything will be the same as before, except cheaper, possibly free. All they will ever have to pay is a nominal co-payment for office visits.

Health care practitioners address this problem by communicating plan rules with their patients from the start of the relationship. They manage their patients' expectations, telling them what to expect, what they can and cannot do in seeking treatment, and generally how the new system works. In most cases, it lowers expectations to more realistic levels.

"The four questions every refractive surgery patient wants answered," says James Colgain, O.D., Fairfax, VA, "are 'Is it safe? Am I a candidate? What results can I expect? Why optometry, which surgeon, and which laser center?' Although each patient may not ask any one of these particular questions directly, I have found that all questions can be placed in one of these four categories. Part of managing expectations is to be sure to answer these questions in your preoperative counseling, even before the patient brings them up."[6]

Generate realistic expectations about refractive surgery, says Paul A. Blaze, O.D., F.A.O., Huntington Beach, CA. "Think of yourself as a patient advocate. Make sure your patient understands the 'real' outcome numbers and knows he may not end up with 20/20 vision. I demonstrate a 20/40 result and make patients aware that this is sufficient to pass a driver's test."[7]

Perry Binder, M.D., San Diego, CA, goes a step further. "In my experience," he says, "the most important LASIK [laser in situ keratomileusis] case to *eliminate* is the patient whose expectations are higher than the outcomes achieved with the average surgical procedure. If patients want a guarantee of surgical results or the same vision currently enjoyed with their gas-permeable contact lenses, then I suggest they reconsider surgery."[8]

On the subject of fitting presbyopes with soft-multifocals, Joe Schwallie, O.D., M.S., Toledo, OH, says, "I educate patients on what to expect. Sometimes patients have the wrong or even unrealistic expectations. Presbyopic patients always experience a compromise, regardless of which type of correction you choose. I tell patients to expect successful vision for about 90% of their daily activities. I identify demanding tasks to uncover the potential for unrealistic expectations. Demanding tasks may limit success during that activity and patients need to know this. I also make sure patients have realistic expectations about the time commitment for success. I explain they will likely return for more than one visit, and they will likely wear more than one pair of lenses before they are happy with their vision. I tell them not to be discouraged if the lenses don't work out on the first try."[9]

104 Perform as promised

- A receptionist calls to remind a patient of his 5 o'clock appointment the following day, but when he arrives punctually, has to wait 20 minutes before being seen.
- An optometrist tells patients of her "24/7 availability" for emergencies, but when called on a weekend, she cannot be reached.
- A patient is promised her glasses on Friday but does not get them until the following week.

Have you had similar disappointments? For example, have you ordered an urgently needed item from a distributor, been told it would be shipped immediately, and then received the wrong item? Or learned the price on the invoice was higher than the one you were quoted on the phone?

Follow-through is abysmal today, and the reasons for that vary. Organizations are understaffed or cutting costs or bogged down by delays they didn't anticipate. Whatever the cause, the result is the same: disappointed and sometimes angry customers, who seldom complain but, in many cases, take their business elsewhere.

ACTION STEPS

Don't make promises you cannot keep, and don't let your staff do so either. Make an extra effort to be on time for appointments, deliver eyewear when promised, return phone calls when you say you will, and provide the quality care and service stated in your practice mission statement.

Most patient complaints stem from poorly managed expectations. Don't waste time trying to exceed patient expectations if you and your staff lack a foolproof system for the basics: delivering *what* you promise, *when* you promise.

Make it an unforgivable sin in your practice to make promises that you do not keep. Consultant Murray Raphel uses the palindromic acronym *D.W.Y.P.Y.W.D.*, which means the same thing backward as it does forward: "Do What You Promised You Would Do."[10]

105   Your top 50

Do you know the identity of the 50 best patients in your practice? Those who have been in the practice the longest? Who bring their entire families to you? Make the most referrals? Spend the most on services, prescription lenses, and eyewear?

Does your staff know them?

Imagine this scenario: one of the top 50 calls your practice, identifies herself, requests an appointment, and is asked by receptionist, "Are you a patient here?"

ACTION STEP

Hold a staff meeting to decide the top 50 patients in your practice, using whatever criteria you think relevant. If you have a really large practice, go for the top 100. If smaller, target the top 20. These are your practice's "movers and shakers."

Keep a list at the front desk. Put an easy-to-spot code on their record or computer file, and give these patients extra-special treatment at every opportunity. Juggle your schedule if necessary to arrange appointments at their convenience, or come in early or stay late to accommodate them. Go to whatever lengths necessary to give them the best possible service. See them on time. Provide personalized attention.

REALITY CHECK

In the best of all worlds, every patient deserves VIP treatment. The peaks and valleys of most practices make that difficult, however, so start with the top 50.

106 Bond patients to your practice

What accounts for patient loyalty, especially in these highly competitive, cost-conscious times? One of the factors frequently mentioned by patients themselves is "they treat you like a friend, not just a number." Obvious? Perhaps, but many offices fail to make a united effort to really do it.

FROM THE SUCCESS FILES

Here is one of the ways this *bonding* of patients is accomplished in the office of Howard L. Kletter, D.D.S., and Paul Baron, D.D.S., Garden City, NY.

Known as the *Personal Note Screen*, it is available at any of the ten computer terminals located throughout Dr. Kletter's office. What it displays is personal information about each patient: family members' names, hobbies, upcoming events such as graduation or vacation, or perhaps a recent event, such as a birth in the family. Such information is gleaned from conversations with patients during office visits (or from reading the hometown newspaper) and then entered into their records.

The office policy is that before speaking with a patient, everyone brings up his or her Personal Note Screen on the computer and scans it. It takes only seconds and changes the entire polarity of a conversation with a patient.

"What it does," Dr. Kletter told me, "is help bring back some of the warmth we lost as our practice grew and our staff became larger."

107 Stay connected to your patients

"It's a growing problem among optometrists," writes John Murphy, Senior Editor of the *Review of Optometry*. "Refractive surgery patients disappear some time after their follow-up care, rarely to reappear in their optometrists' offices."

FROM THE SUCCESS FILES

Wallace Ryne, O.D., F.A.A.O., Southlake, TX, started escorting all his refractive surgery patients to the laser center, eventually going into the surgical suite and assisting with the procedure itself. It's the best way, the only way, he says, to remain connected to the patient throughout the refractive surgery process.

"In return, patients stay connected to you. They remain in your appointment book. Usually don't disappear after their follow-up care is done. And best of all," says Dr. Ryne, "when they talk about LASIK, they talk about you."[11]

Paul A. Blaze, O.D., F.A.A.O., Huntington Beach, CA, concurs. "Be there on the day of surgery," he says. "Many patients are comforted by my presence. Speaking with their accompanying family or friends about the procedure and having them view the procedure has resulted in many collateral referrals to my office."

"Then, do the 1-day post-op," says Dr. Blaze. "This is where you'll see the 'wow' factor. Being present for this will bond you to your enthusiastic patient. I go so far as to give patients my cell phone number in case they have more questions and I call them in the evening after their surgery. Reinforce that you're also pleased with the results. Remind them that these results are in line with your pre-op expectations."[7]

---

108 Secrets of award-winning service

It is always a treat to stay at a Ritz-Carlton hotel: Fresh flowers are everywhere, there are luxurious terry cloth bathrobes in each guest's room, and there are countless amenities. Most noteworthy and universally appreciated by travelers, however, is the outstanding service.

The Ritz-Carlton Hotel Company has *twice* won the prestigious Malcolm Baldridge National Quality Award, which was established by Congress in 1987 to promote quality management.

What's their secret?

A 3-day orientation introduces every Ritz-Carlton employee to the following core values:

1. "Ritz-Carlton Hotel is a place where the genuine care and comfort of our guests is our highest mission."
2. "At the Ritz-Carlton, we are ladies and gentlemen serving ladies and gentlemen."
3. "The three steps of service expected of every employee are a warm and sincere greeting using the guest's name; anticipation and compliance with guests' needs; and a fond farewell."

Ritz-Carlton trains employees with a thorough orientation followed by on-the-job training, then job certification. If an employee detects guest dissatisfaction, for example, he or she is empowered to break away from the routine and take immediate positive action, to "move heaven and earth" to remedy the situation. Or, the employee can call on any other employee to assist. The Ritz-Carlton refers to this as "lateral service" and encourages it.

Other Ritz-Carlton training basics include these service standards that apply whether someone is making beds, washing dishes, or selling rooms:

- Smile—we are on stage.
- Assume responsibility for uncompromising levels of cleanliness.
- Any employee who receives a guest complaint "owns" the complaint. "This means if a guest tells a housekeeper the TV doesn't work, the housekeeper must find an engineer to fix the set and report back to the guest that the problem has been solved. This gets complaints resolved incredibly quickly and gives customers another reason for being delighted with our service." [12]
- Use the proper vocabulary with our guests (words like "good morning," "certainly," "I'll be happy to," and "my pleasure").
- Always maintain positive eye contact.
- Escort guests, rather than pointing out directions to another area of the hotel.
- Be an ambassador of your hotel in and outside of the workplace.
- Always talk positively. No negative comments.

"Although many hotel companies have rigorous training programs, the Ritz-Carlton is in a class by itself," says M. L. Smith, professor of hospitality marketing at the University of Nevada's College of Hotel Administration. "They have figured out what guests want in a hotel," he adds, "and learned how to exceed their expectations."[13]

109 Be good on the basics

"The most important thing," says J. W. Marriott, founder of the Marriott Corporation, "is to serve the hot food hot and the cold food cold."

He is talking, of course, about the importance of *basics*, and it is as true about optometric service as it is about food service. You may have sunk a fortune into the design and construction of your office and have the newest and best equipment on the market, but if you and your staff do not deliver on what patients consider the *basics* of good service, you've missed the boat, big time.

What are the basics? They are the fundamental things that decide whether or not patients pay their bills cheerfully and promptly, remain loyal to your practice, and refer others to you.

Marriott identified its basics by analyzing the results of a comprehensive guest survey. They learned that guests' intent to return rests on five critical factors: everything is clean and works; check-in is hassle free; staff is friendly and helpful; problems are resolved quickly; breakfast is served on time.

When Marriott fails to deliver on these basic expectations, guests have an unsatisfactory stay at a Marriott hotel. No amount of mints on the pillow will bring back a guest who had to wait 30 minutes to check in, whose bathroom was dirty, and whose breakfast was overcooked and late in coming.

ACTION STEPS

Decide with your staff what basic services matter most to your patients. Use the following statement and fill in the blanks: "Nothing else matters if we don't _____ or aren't _____."

This is one of the exercises I have seminar audiences do. Answers have included: readily available for emergencies; on time for appointments; nice to patients; have a meticulously clean office; answer patients' questions; deliver glasses when promised.

Be good on the basics and patients tolerate almost anything else. Screw up on the basics and nothing else matters. Patients will not return. Period.

FROM THE SUCCESS FILES

"One of the basics considered most important," says Erwin Jay, O.D., Richmond Heights, OH, "is 'Whatever else you do for patients, at the very least, satisfy their chief complaint.'" Obvious? "Many of the patients we see in our offices tell us that their former doctor did not satisfy their chief complaint."[14]

---

110 Decide what you want to be famous for

It could be any one of 101 things that differentiate your practice; set it apart from others in the community; and, most importantly, appeal to your target population.

For example, Midwest Express Airlines wants to be famous for "The best care in the air," its signature statement in all advertising. They walk their talk: Coach passengers are treated as though they are flying first class. No middle seats. The seats are larger than average, leather, and comfortable. Full meals are served on china along with complimentary wine or champagne and chocolate chip cookies (freshly baked on board). The flight attendants are invariably friendly. In a commodity-like industry, Midwest Express is a non-commodity player with a very loyal following.

The positioning strategy of Federal Express is based on a simple promise: "When it absolutely, positively has to be there overnight."

Larry Rosenthal, D.D.S., New York, NY, is widely known for his expertise in cosmetic dentistry and has created many "celebrity smiles." His commitment to patients is "Five-Star Service. Five-Star Product."

The goal of Lawrence J. Jacobs, O.D., Highlands Ranch, CO, is to impress patients in three ways: office ambiance, instruments, and professionalism.[15]

These lofty aspirations set the stage. Simplify the task of day-to-day operation. Make it easier for everyone to stay focused and, as the politicians say, "on message."

111 It starts at the top

Those qualities for which you want your practice to be famous are not going to just "happen" on their own.

In his book, *The Will to Manage* (McGraw-Hill, 1996) Marvin Bower says it is a manager's responsibility to spell out for employees "the way we do things around here." Bower's implied assumption is that unless you tell people what you want them to do and how you want them to do it, you have no right to expect them to infer by some mysterious means just what you have in mind.

FROM THE SUCCESS FILES

The following letter, sent to new employees of a physician's office, illustrates the principle Bower describes previously:

Dear Chris,

Welcome aboard! We are pleased to welcome you to our health care team and want you to be part of our continued success. To that end, I want to take a minute to reiterate the reason for our being here. If you remember these principles, I guarantee that you will succeed at your job and reap the rewards. Remember

- *Above all, you are here to serve patients. Each of us is. The patient signs our paycheck.*
- *Our practice is built on medical quality and patient service. Strive for uncompromising quality in every phase of your job. Efficiency, precision, and attention to detail are all part of serving the patient.*
- *Every person who walks through our door—patient, postman, management consultant, sales representative—is an honored guest. Each of us is an ambassador of goodwill. We want you to astonish them with your courtesy, concern, and genuine caring for their comfort and well being.*
- *Know your patients. Greet them by name and with a smile as soon as they walk through our door. Let them know you appreciate them.*

> - *Handle any patient problems or complaints with the utmost courtesy, concern, and respect. Remember, the patient is our boss.*
>
> *In short, we're all working for the same goals. If we apply these principles of patient satisfaction and professional excellence to our particular skills everyday, there's no stopping us.*
>
> *Again, I welcome you to our office and look forward to working with you for a long and rewarding future.*
>
> *Sincerely,*

Benefits of Such a Letter

- Establishes, in writing, the *priorities* of your practice
- Spells out in a simple, straightforward manner what's expected of everyone
- Provides a baseline against which future performance can be evaluated

112 Follow-up phone calls

A "moment of truth" that may have clinical significance is the phone call after an office visit for an emergency such as a corneal abrasion or treatment for conjunctivitis. The purpose? To see how the patient is doing.

ACTION STEP

Follow-up phone calls can be made from the office (between patients), on the way home from a car phone, or from your home. They need not be time consuming.

Explain the purpose of the call by saying at the start, "I'm just between appointments (or "on my way home" or "about to sit down to dinner") and I was thinking of you. How are you feeling?"

Occasionally, patients have discomfort that they had not expected or perhaps, more discomfort than they expected—with varying degrees of concern about what it means.

The situation may just call for reassurance, a reminder of (previously given) home-care instructions, an adjustment in medication, or other special instructions depending on the symptoms.

In such cases, there is an opportunity to turn even this highly positive "moment of truth" into a *truly memorable* one—by telephoning an anxious patient a *second time* later the same day or evening to see if the home-care instructions, medication, or just the passage of time has improved the situation.

Follow-up phone calls occasionally uncover situations that need further attention. More frequently, they give patients "peace of mind" about what they're experiencing and evidence of your genuine interest in them.

REALITY CHECK

In today's impersonal, take-a-number, have-a-seat health care environment, such calls make a highly favorable, lasting impression on patients.

113   Welcome complaints

Some staff members think of patient complaints as *annoyances*. It makes more sense to regard them as an *opportunity* to learn what upsets patients, correct the problem, retain their goodwill, and possibly impress them.

REALITY CHECK

Current research shows that only 4% of dissatisfied patients even bother to complain, at least to the person who either caused or could remedy the problem. Many consider it futile and a waste of time. Some are afraid of being labeled a "complainer." So, those who *do* are, in essence, doing you a favor.

Deftly handled, complaints can be neutralized and possibly made into a positive experience. Ineptly handled, they can "lose" a patient.

114 Hard-learned lessons about complaints

- Patients who would not dream of confronting *you* with a complaint may easily direct their anger to *your staff.*
- Make sure your staff understands the importance of patient retention. Some employees honestly believe that loyalty requires them to *defend* the practice at all costs and never give in to a complaining patient.
- A sign in the staff lounge of one office reads "Never let a patient go away mad—without first seeing the doctor—unless it was the *doctor* who made the patient mad."
- Always assume patients have a legitimate complaint. Even if they don't, *they* think they do, so hear them out. Don't interrupt. When patients tell you what's bothering them, show concern. If appropriate, take notes. Such actions show you're interested and paying attention. If a patient has overreacted to the situation or exaggerated the complaint, he or she will become calmer simply by seeing you are sympathetic and responsive.
- Thank patients for speaking up. If you respond negatively when patients tell you or your staff things you don't want to hear, you'll stop getting the feedback you need to improve.
- Concede before you contend. Agree with what the patient says before responding. For example, "I can understand why you are upset. I'd feel the same way if I were in your shoes." Patients tend to be more reasonable and receptive to what you have to say when they realize you're not being defensive or argumentative about the situation.
- When voicing complaints about poor service, patients are not interested in hearing lengthy explanations of your problems.
- "Trivializing a patient's complaint," says Larry K. Wan, O.D., Campbell, CA, "is a surefire way to lose that patient. The response from anyone in your office to a patient complaint should be: 'Let me see what I can do to help you.'"[16]
- Whenever possible, do what you can to resolve the situation in the patient's favor. Admit your mistake. Apologize. If that falls short, stop and say, "I really feel badly about what happened. What can

we do to correct the problem?" The patient's tone usually changes immediately. Many forgive and forget. If the patient has a reasonable request, agree to it—immediately. If such measures are required only occasionally, the costs will be minimal and you'll generate incalculable goodwill.

- "One of the most important things that we train staff members to do is service recovery," says Don Robinson, senior vice president, resort operations, Walt Disney World Co. "That's when you walk into a situation and you can tell that something has gone wrong— and you do whatever it takes to fix the problem. That's also an opportunity for what we call a 'magic moment.'"[1]
- "The rule is to take responsibility and fix the problem," says John Bruns, general manager of the Ritz-Carlton in Cleveland, OH. "And remember that speed counts. Don't question the customer; just fix the problem, and fix it fast."[17]
- Tom Peters has observed, "A well-handled complaint usually breeds more loyalty than existed before the incident occurred."

115 Beware of backlash

The advent of the Internet means that patients have more ways than ever to vent their dissatisfaction. Case in point: http://www.surgicaleyes.org, a Web site that exists (in their words) "to help people who have had unsuccessful LASIK, PRK, RK, AK, ALK, or other elective refractive surgeries that resulted in debilitating complications."

Another Web site that contains intensely compelling reports of patient suffering and utter devastation is self-descriptive: http://www.lasikdisaster.com.

"With tools like the Internet making it easier than ever for dissatisfied customers to be heard," says Alexa K. Apallas, "one well-publicized complaint can leave hundreds of potential customers with a negative impression."[18]

116 Strive for patient loyalty

"One of the biggest mistakes we've made in the past," says Tim Banker, D.V.M., Greensboro, NC, "is to take loyal clients for granted while spinning our wheels trying to get new clients. We now let loyal clients know how much we appreciate them."

There are many benefits (beyond the obvious) of having loyal patients:

- Loyal patients, by definition, have more trust in the recommendations made by optometrists, opticians, and staff members. They tend to come in more often and spend more per visit.
- Loyal patients tend to be more tolerant of minor problems, delays, and the like.
- Loyal patients are the most vocal in telling others about the quality of care and service they received.
- Revenue grows as a result of repeat visits, purchases, and referrals.
- Costs decline as a result of the efficiencies of seeing "experienced" patients who require less paperwork and explanations.
- Costs also decline as the need for advertising and practice promotion decrease. (It costs 5 times more to acquire a new patient than it does to retain an existing one.)
- Employee retention increases because of job pride and satisfaction, which in turn creates a loop that reinforces patient loyalty and further reduces costs as hiring and training costs decrease and productivity rises.
- As costs go down and revenues go up, *profitability* increases.

117 Acknowledge loyal patients

- 10–30% of optometric patients are fiercely loyal and not likely to switch to another office.

- 25–50% are more or less inclined to stay with the same doctor of optometry. Unlike the first grouping, they can be, and often are, "lured" away by competitors.
- Finally, 10–25% really do not care where they go or whom they see. They tend to view eye exams, contact lenses, and "glasses" as *commodities* and select them strictly on price or convenience or because a provider is listed in a directory from a managed-care plan.

ACTION STEP

Let loyal patients know how much you appreciate them, and strive as a team to upgrade more middle-of-the-road patients into that fiercely loyal category. For example, tell a long-term patient of record, "As I was reviewing your chart this morning, I noted that you've been with our practice for more than 15 years. Thank you for your confidence in us. We've really enjoyed having you in our practice."

Say it, of course, in your own words. Or, write it if that's more comfortable. As an old saying goes, people love doing business with those who appreciate their business.

118 Retention versus loyalty

Patient retention is not the same thing as patient loyalty. If you're the only optometrist in town, you'll retain your patients. Suppose, however, other practices open up in your area—will your patients remain loyal?

Loyalty implies a *choice*. It's a very important distinction.

"Core service doesn't generate loyalty," says Stephanie A. Busty, a training specialist at New York City's Beth Israel Hospital. "It's getting the service up to extraordinary levels. We want to exceed expectations. We want to knock their socks off."[19]

119 Keep contact lens patients loyal to your practice

"With the emergence of various Internet sites and 1-800 numbers, not to mention the impact of managed care," writes Deepak Gupta, O.D.,

Stamford, CT, "how can you keep contact lens patients loyal to your practice?" Among his suggestions: "Ship lenses directly to your patients. Most manufacturers offer this service free as long as you order a 6-month or year's supply. Some of the benefits of direct shipping are

- Patients will order multiple boxes of contact lenses instead of one or two, increasing your revenue.
- Patients must pay for their contact lenses up front, decreasing your accounts receivable.
- Your staff will not have to receive the shipments, call patients when they arrive, hold the contact lenses until the patients can pick them up, and complete the transactions when they do. This can be a tremendous timesaver.
- Patients are buying a 6-month or year's supply of contact lenses so they have less incentive to search for them elsewhere."[20]

REALITY CHECK

"I think direct shipments of contact lenses are the primary care optometrist's only alternative to losing patients to Web- or phone-based lens replacement services," says technology consultant Rick Potvin, O.D. "It provides the convenience that is required by the public, and keeps the doctor in the loop."[21]

120 Hard-learned lessons about patient expectations

- "The practitioner who is able to fully understand the expectations of the patient at each encounter," say Stuart Rothman, O.D., Harry Kaplan, O.D., and Craig Hisaka, O.D., M.P.H., "will be the one who establishes a long-term relationship with the patient."[22]
- The obvious secret of exceeding patients' expectations: Under-promise. Over-deliver.
- "Achieving a high level of patient satisfaction," says Stephen Cohen, O.D., Scottsdale, AZ, "has helped me to successfully increase patient and staff loyalty, staff morale, referrals, efficiency, and productivity, while also decreasing staff turnover and the likelihood of malpractice suits."[23]

- "Service is just a day-in, day-out, ongoing, never-ending, unremitting, persevering, compassionate type of activity," says Leon Gorman, president of L. L. Bean Inc.
- "Clients do us a favor by deciding to come to us—not the other way around," says Joyce M. Hansen, practice manager of the Northampton Veterinary Clinic in Northampton, MA.
- "There is a special feeling that washes over most people when they interact with another human being to whom they are handing money. That feeling is entitlement. They want to be served. They think they *deserve* it."[24]
- "In southern California, where computer discount stores hang on to solvency by slashing costs and getting by on the flimsiest of margins, a company called ComputerLand Technology Resources flourishes despite its higher prices," says Eric Anderson, M.D., San Diego, CA. "A plaque on the wall, displayed where every employee can read it, carries the corporate motto. It says, in part:

> *We believe business will continue to go where it is invited and remain where it is appreciated.*
> *We believe reputations will continue to be made by many acts and lost by one.*
> *We believe trust, not tricks, will keep clients loyal.*
> *We believe the extra mile has no traffic jams.*[25]

Notes

1. McCauley L. How May I Help You? *Fast Company*, March 2000, 93–126.
2. Peters T, Austin N. *A Passion for Excellence.* New York: Random House, 1985.
3. *Yankelovich Monitor*, July 23, 2001.
4. Wood N. So You Want a Revolution. *Incentive*, June 1998, 41–47.
5. Albrecht K, Bradford, LJ. *The Service Advantage: How to Identify and Fulfill Customer Needs.* Homewood, IL: Dow Jones-Irwin, 1990.
6. Colgain J. Managing Patient Expectations with LASIK. http://www.refractivesource.com.
7. Blaze PA. Will LASIK Co-Management Fees Dry Up? *Optometric Management*, March 2000, 94–97.
8. Binder PS. Identifying the "Wrong" LASIK Candidates. http://www.sightstreet.com, July 11, 2001.

9. Schwallie J. Successful Multi-focal Contact Lens Fitting. *Contact Lens Spectrum*, June 2001, 12S–15S.

10. Raphel M, Raphel N. *Up the Loyalty Ladder: Turning Sometime Customers into Full-Time Advocates of Your Business.* New York: HarperBusiness, 1995.

11. Murphy M. Go into the O.R., Come out with a Loyal Patient. *Review of Optometry*, October 2001, 56–58,61.

12. Marriott WJ Jr. The Marriott System: To Delight Customers Again and Again. *Bottom Line/Business*, June 1998, 3–4.

13. McDowell E. Ritz-Carlton's Keys to Good Service. *New York Times*, March 31, 1993, D1,5.

14. Jay E. Guaranteed Practice Builders, Volume 1. Richmond Heights, OH, 1992.

15. Eisenberg JS. Rocky Mountain Doctor Looks to Scale New Heights. *Review of Optometry*, March 2000, 71–72,74,76.

16. Wan LK. Strategies for Better Patient Retention. *Optometric Management*, September 2000, 3s–8s.

17. Lessons to Be Learned from "Gold Standards." *Practice Marketing and Management*, October 1998, 135,137.

18. Appalls AK. The Power of Public Opinion. *Customer Relationship Management*, May 2000, 122.

19. Fein EB. To Compete, Hospitals Get Hoteliers' Service Lessons. *New York Times*, July 24, 1995, B1,B6.

20. Gupta D. How to Be the Must-See O.D. *Optometric Management*, April 2001.

21. Byrne J. Practitioner-Based Web Sites: Another Way to Provide the Highest Level of Care. *Primary Care Optometry News*, September 2001, 12.

22. Rothman S, Kaplan H, Hisaka C. Patient Communication. *Business Aspects of Optometry*, edited by JG Classé, C Hisaka, DH Lakin, et al. (eds). Boston: Butterworth–Heinemann, 1997.

23. Cohen S. Unlocking the Secrets to Exceptional Patient Satisfaction. *Optometric Management*, August 2001, 45–46,48,50,53.

24. Steinhauer J. Would a Clerk by Any Other Name Measure Your Feet? *New York Times*, March 30, 1997.

25. Anderson E. We Need to Get Better at "Customer Service." *Medical Economics*, April 12, 1999, 275–276.

7

Hard-Learned Lessons about Fees

121 Price isn't everything

Studies of consumer behavior indicate that only 13% of people make buying decisions based *strictly on price*. The consumers in this small group, either because of economic circumstances or because they don't know better, always look for the lowest price. That means 87% of people consider price, but *also* look for quality, good service, convenience, a personal relationship, and more from their service providers.

Considering the buying potential of each group, does it make sense to gear your practice and fee structure to the price-conscious 13% of the population? You may drown in overhead costs trying to keep prices low enough to suit them. And, by definition, they will leave your practice if they can find lower prices elsewhere.

You may be thinking that more than 13% of your community is price conscious. Perhaps so, but even if you double this number, that leaves 74% of people who are interested in factors besides cost—still a sizable target population for your practice. If you tripled the figure to 39%, you could still target 61% of the population as prospective patients—more than you and your present staff could handle.

You can't be all things to all people, so why not provide the quality of care, personal service, convenience, and one-to-one relationships that meet the needs of the 87% to whom price is not everything?

HARD-LEARNED LESSON

"There's nothing wrong with competing on price," says Robert B. Tucker, author of *Win the Value Revolution* (Career Press, 1995), "but if being the 'low price leader' in your market isn't your full-bore, dead-on strategy, then flirting with price competition could become your firm's eventual death certificate."

REALITY CHECK

If price were everything, supermarket shelves would be filled with generic products priced lower than their branded counterparts. As it is, generic products account for only a small fraction of supermarket sales.

122 Put fees in proper perspective

Which of these cards looks bigger: the one with the word *Value* or the one with the word *Price*?

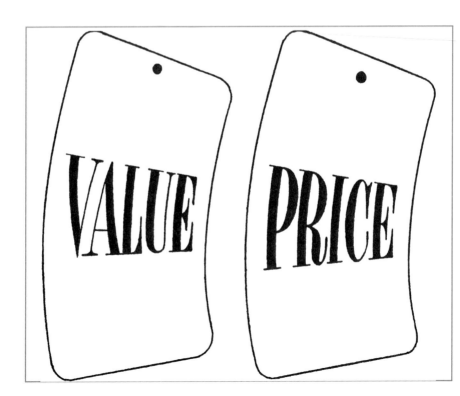

Most people say the card with the word *Price* looks bigger. Actually, the cards are the same size. The Price card appears larger because the eyes tend to focus on the center of the picture where the short side of the Value card is compared to the long side of the Price card.

Most people make "buying decisions" based on these two factors, *value* and *price*. When a product or service has unique features or benefits that set it apart from others, it has *added value* and commands a *premium price* or *fee*. If such benefits and features are meaningful to people (and they can afford them), they will choose the quality product or service.

Conversely, if people perceive a product or service as a *commodity*, alike in all respects to competing products and services, then *cost* becomes the chief consideration. It makes sense: Why should people pay extra for something they don't value?

To put your fees in proper perspective, you'll want to reverse the previous picture. Make *value* the focus of attention.

Differentiating your practice, providing value-added services, explaining the benefits of premium lens options, *and* letting patients

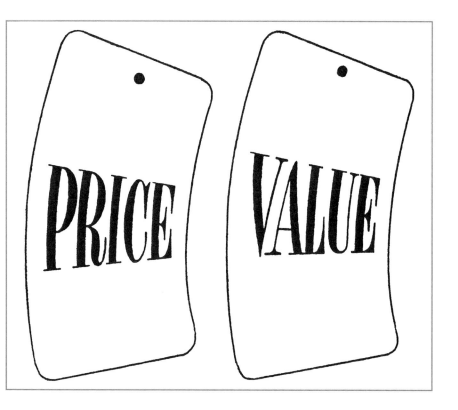

know the particulars, helps them see the entire picture and put fees in proper perspective.

A common mistake is to assume that *value* and *price* mean the same thing to patients. They don't. Price is price; value is the total experience.

FROM THE SUCCESS FILES

"Many practitioners charge an additional fee for routine annual contact lens exams," says Stephen Cohen, O.D., Scottsdale, AZ. "Often, patients question this fee—particularly when their contact lens prescription hasn't changed. An in-office form such as the following can help remedy this potential area of contention."

"To us, the items seem routine," adds Dr. Cohen. "However, patients don't always know what differentiates one type of exam from another and often, one provider from another."[1]

We're dedicated to providing you with the most comprehensive contact lens care possible. To ensure your long-term success, we will

- Evaluate your visual acuity with your current contact lenses
- Determine any contact lens prescription change
- Assess the fit of your current contact lenses
- Microscopically evaluate the health of the front surface of your eyes
- Measure the shape of the front surface of your eyes
- Review the results of this evaluation and discuss available options with you

As one of the largest contact lens practices in the state, we provide consultation services to major contact lens manufacturers and typically receive new products before they're available to eye care providers. This allows us to keep you informed of the latest advances in contact lens technology.

---

123 Economic realities of discounted fees

Have you been tempted to lower your fees to jump-start a sluggish practice on the assumption that 70–80% of your usual fees is better than nothing? It is a bad move.

REALITY CHECK

The discounting of fees requires a *huge increase* of patients just to maintain your previous level of profitability, let alone exceed it.

Assume a solo practitioner performs 2,500 eye examinations a year at an average fee of $100 and an overhead of 60%. (Your numbers may be higher or lower—the algorithm is the same.) In this scenario, the gross income (from examinations only) is $250,000; the overhead is $150,000, leaving a net profit of $100,000 and a healthy profit margin of 40%.

If the average fee of $100 is now discounted by 20%, the net profit drops to $50,000—*half of what it was previously*! (2,500 exams at $80 each = $200,000 less the [same] overhead of $150,000.) Most significant, this now reduces the profit margin to just 25%.

The following table illustrates the disastrous effects of various fee discounts on net income:

Impact of Discounted Fees on Net Income (Assuming an Overhead of 60%)

Discount (%)	Production ($)	Gross Income ($)	Overhead ($)	Profit ($)	Reduction in Net Income (%)
No discount	100	100	60	40	0
20	100	80	60	20	50
30	100	70	60	10	75
40	100	60	60	0	100

To return the practice to its previous level of profitability ($100,000) requires a minimum of *5,000* comprehensive exams (*twice as many as before*) at $80 each to now reach $400,000, assuming the profit margin remains at 25%. To make that happen, you'll need to work faster, and most likely, longer hours than you did previously.

124   No surprises

The two-word formula to reduce complaints about fees is *no surprises*.

"Anyone who makes appointments must find out the name of the patient's vision or health plan when the patient calls to schedule his or her visit," says Neil B. Gailmard, O.D., M.B.A., Munster, IN. "You want patients to know and accept your policies before they show up. If the patient has a plan you accept, your staff should obtain authorization of benefits before the appointment. If the patient has a plan that isn't on your approved list, the receptionist should tell him or her that your office doesn't accept the benefits directly, but the patient can submit the claim. State the exam fee over the phone and inform the patient that payment is due at the time of service. While this may seem like a tough approach, if these terms are not acceptable, you don't want the patient to make an appointment."[2]

"You may think it's unprofessional to discuss money up front," says Deepak Gupta, O.D., Stamford, CT, "but I think it's much less professional to have a patient in the waiting room who's angry because he wasn't told about fees or insurance plans in advance. If you're going to scare a patient away because of your fees or because you don't accept his insurance, do it before he walks into your office and makes a scene. The only scenario that's worse is when a patient refuses to pay for services he's already received because no one explained the fees ahead of time."[3]

125 What does your staff think of your fees?

What your staff members think of your fees can influence patient acceptance and your professional image—for better or for worse. If, for example, they believe your fees are high, they may unintentionally undermine your fees and lead patients to believe they're overpaying for your services. How? If a patient complains about a fee (or a fee increase) and they give a "what-can-I-do-about-it" shrug, it could be construed as tacit agreement. Voicing those same words would be deadly. Even saying nothing at such times can come across badly.

To test the waters, ask each staff member: "Do you think our fees are about right? Too high? Too low?" See what they say.

If their answers indicate they think fees are on the high side, the next step is to educate your staff as to why you charge what you do. Be prepared, however, for some surprises—at both extremes. I frequently encounter staff members who believe the fees in their office are "too low." They obviously value the doctor's time, skill, knowledge, and investment in education and equipment more than the doctor does.

---

126 How to handle complaints about fees

Do patients ever complain about fees? Ask for a discount? Compare your fees (or prices) with lower fees (or prices) advertised by others? Here is one way to respond:

"Our fees are based on a number of factors: the time and level of skill involved, the number of services provided, the caliber of people who work with me, our facilities and equipment, the continuing education of all staff members, our laboratory costs, and the quality of materials used. If we were to reduce fees, we'd have to leave something out, and frankly I don't know what to eliminate without compromising the quality of what we do."

No need to use these words as such: They're just a track to run on; a way to give patients something to think about other than cost.

This explanation is even more meaningful if patients already know about each of these components of your fee. Office tours, practice brochures, Web site descriptions, continuing education notices (Chapter 5), itemized bills, and explanations of the services that you and your staff provide, all help make patients aware and appreciative of what's involved.

FROM THE SUCCESS FILES

"Our patients understand the difference between our refractive surgical practice and the discount laser center," says Barry Eiden, O.D., F.A.A.O., Chicago, IL. "We emphasize

- Our long experience.
- Our involvement in research.
- Our positions as advisory board members and consultants to surgical companies and organizations.

- Our comprehensive care program (extended follow-up care and complimentary enhancements or modifications) versus the limited postoperative care and charges for enhancement at discount centers.
- Most of all, we emphasize our unbiased viewpoint. We provide all types of refractive care (glasses, contact lenses, and refractive surgery) with equal expertise and emphasis. Our recommendations are based on what we sincerely feel is in the patient's best interest."[4]

127 How important are fees?

At a recent seminar I conducted for accountants, I met a middle-aged practitioner whose specialty was agricultural economics. He told me that several years before, he had suffered a major heart attack, spent close to 2 months in the hospital, and then additional time at home before returning to work on a part-time basis. His physician's advice was succinct and no-nonsense: Cut your workload and client list *in half*, or you are not going to make it!

Sensing the life/death consequences of the situation, this hard-working accountant heeded his doctor's advice. He sent a form letter to all of his tax and audit clients explaining the situation, the need to cut back, and (with an eye on keeping his practice economically afloat) the necessity to *double his fees*!

He added that he recognized this would create a hardship for some of his clients and would understand if they needed to transfer their records and any future work to another practitioner. He ended the letter by asking his clients to please call his office with further instructions.

How did his clients react to the letter? More than 90% called to say they would remain with him.

Obviously, a number of factors accounted for this allegiance. The question, however, remains: How important are fees? The answer is, probably less than you think.

REALITY CHECK

You offer patients an experience in your practice that is unique to your practice. Although there are many highly competent optometrists, your chairside manner, personality, and style of running your practice are unique to you as an individual. If patients want you, they will pay your fee.

128 Hard-learned lessons about fees

- I have yet to meet the optometrist whose profitability dropped as a result of a reasonable fee increase.
- A 10–15% fee differential is almost never the reason that patients change from one practice to another. In many cases, their decisions are based on emotional factors including trust, confidence, rapport, likeability, and perceived value.
- Make *clinical* decisions for patients—not *economic* decisions. There is no way you can ascertain what patients are willing to pay or can afford. Recommend what's best for patients. Let *them* decide if that's what they want.
- Charge private-pay patients for what you do based on your overhead, time, and expertise. *Especially* your expertise. "Clinical expertise," says Jack Schaeffer, O.D., Birmingham, AL, "is the most significant income-producing asset in your practice."[5]
- "You're losing money if you don't bill for the time you spend on decision-making, monitoring, and follow-up while managing medical cases," says Rebecca Wartman, O.D., Asheville, NC.[6]
- "Many of our patients have had contact lens failures in the past," says Kenneth A. Lebow, O.D., F.A.A.O., Virginia Beach, VA, "and they don't want to buy materials if they can't wear the lenses. We're up front with these individuals. We tell them, 'You don't have to buy any materials until we know you'll be successful, but you'll have to pay for the time I spend with you.' Patients are usually very receptive to that, and we've been successful in presenting our fees on that basis."[7]

- You pride yourself on excellence, a fact reflected in your fee structure. To maintain your high standards, you cannot discount your services *or* compete on the basis of price with optometrists whose niche includes bargain-hunting patients.
- Bargain-hunting patients are the worst source of referrals. They refer only other bargain-hunters.
- "Cutting prices is usually insanity," says Harvard Business School professor Michael Porter, "if the competition can go as low as you can. You have to find a different competitive tack. Quality becomes central—and so do service and innovation."[8]
- I've seen more practices hurt by fees that were *too low* than I have by fees that were *too high*.
- "Say you've neglected to adjust your fees for several years," says Carol A. Schwartz, O.D., M.B.A., F.A.A.O., Vista, CA, "and find you need to make a 30% increase. Because you've obviously been undercharging, you may have attracted a number of price-sensitive patients. What you'll do is make your fee increase, but inform current patients that they'll continue to pay the old rate as a reward for their loyalty. At the end of a set period, discontinue the courtesy discount. You'll lose some prior patients, but you'll replace them with less price-sensitive individuals who are healthier for your practice."[9]
- "Charge appropriately for your services," says Douglas P. Benoit, O.D., F.A.A.O., Concord, NH. "Consider separating professional fees from material charges and explaining this breakdown so the patient does not perceive the charge as 'just for two contact lenses.' Keep the professional fees higher and the material charges lower. This keeps replacement lens costs lower as well as discourages patients from shopping around once the fitting is complete."[10]
- If you are not already doing so, consider electronic claims submission. "The handwriting is on the wall," says Charles B. Brownlow, O.D., F.A.A.O., executive vice president of the Wisconsin Optometric Association. "Handwritten claims are on the way out. Electronic claims submission has increased efficiency, lowered costs, reduced filing errors, and increased the speed with which claims are processed and providers are reimbursed."[11]
- Low fees (or prices) tend to attract patients who, by definition, are going to leave your practice if they find lower fees (or prices) elsewhere.

- There will always be someone willing to do what you do at a lower fee.
- Resist knocking low-cost competition with the "apples versus oranges" argument. In addition to legal and ethical considerations, it may sound like sour grapes. It is better to acknowledge that your fees are higher. Then explain, if necessary, that the services you and your staff provide require more time and attention to detail than lower fees would allow. The *implication* is that your services are superior.
- Discounting fees devalues optometric services. It also devalues you.
- Patients (like all consumers) tend to relate *quality* to *cost*. "If you pay more, it's probably *worth* more," goes the theory. Obviously, this is only a perception—one that is generally true. Like it or not, many optometrists' reputations for quality are based solely on their fees.
- If you never get complaints about fees, it means either you and your staff are providing high-quality care and first-rate service and your patients think it is worth every penny or you are undercharging.
- It doesn't make sense to provide clinical excellence and charge for mediocrity.
- By the same token, high fees in a shabby, understaffed environment don't work.
- When you raise fees, should you give patients advance notice? Write letters with explanations about escalating costs? Post bulletin board notices? The consensus of optometrists with whom I've spoken is "Just *do* it."
- Remember that if you raise fees, you're under no obligation to maintain them. If there are signs of significant resistance, you can and possibly should reduce fees to their previous levels, but first do the math. Sometimes, less is more.
- "Our practice is definitely not high end in terms of practice location, high tech equipment or in the socioeconomic level of our patients," says Robert B. Sanet, O.D., F.C.O.V.D., Lemon Grove, CA. "However, over the 13 years we have been in partnership, Dr. Carl Hillier and I have raised our fees an average of over 18 percent per year for a total increase of just over 273%. In this period, the number of patients receiving optometric vision therapy at any one time has tripled."[12]
- In all the years I have been surveying optometrists on the subject, I have met only a handful who raised their fees and later regretted it.

REALITY CHECK

Take a long, hard look at your fees. It is no secret that overhead costs in optometric offices have been rising steadily. You need to set realistic fees that enable you to pay a top-notch staff excellent wages, have state-of-the-art equipment and a first-rate office, spend quality time with each patient and not feel pressured to overbook yourself, and, in the final analysis, generate a reasonable profit.

Notes

1. Cohen S. Discovering the Key to Effectively Educating Patients. *Optometric Management,* September 2001, 59–61,64,66.
2. Gailmard NB. Calculate Your Chair Costs in These 5 Easy Steps. *Review of Optometry,* June 1999, 70–74.
3. Gupta D. How to Be the Must-See O.D. *Optometric Management,* April 2001, 7–8.
4. Eiden B. The Proactive Therapeutic Approach. *Optometric Management,* September 2001, 92–96.
5. Schaeffer J. Take a Closer Look at Clinical Exams. *Optometric Management,* June 1994, 21.
6. Wartman R. Profiting with Therapeutics. *Optometric Management,* August 1998, 18S–19S.
7. Lord RW, Oliphant SC, Lebow KA. Strategies to Grow Your Contact Lens Practice. *Optometric Management,* July 2001, 3S–6S.
8. McCormick J, Powell B. Management for the 1990s. *Newsweek,* April 25, 1988, 47.
9. Schwartz CA. Raising Your Fees without Raising the Roof. *Optometric Management,* July 2000, 92–94,144.
10. Benoit DP. Multifocal Contact Lens Update. *Contact Lens Spectrum,* November 2001, 26–31.
11. Brownlow CR. Avoid Potential Filing Fees by Implementing Electronic Claims Submission. *Primary Care Optometry News,* August 2001, 10.
12. Sanet RB. Rationale for Fee Structures. *Developing the Dynamic Vision Therapy Practice,* edited by WB Bleything. Santa Ana, CA: Optometric Extension Program Foundation, 1998, 85–91.

8

The Good, the Bad, and the Ugly

We are all familiar with that part of the retina that is not affected by light and has no sensation of vision, called the *blind spot*. "Blind spots" also occur in the management of a practice when doctors and staff members fail to see the impact their words, actions, office policies, and procedures have on patient satisfaction and loyalty.

One purpose of *marketing research*, the subject of this chapter, is to identify those management "blind spots" to learn the following:

- What you and your staff are doing *right* in your practice
- What, if anything, you are doing *wrong*
- What changes, if any, are needed

129 What's No. 1?

"We spend in the neighborhood of $10 million a year on market research," says J. Willard (Bill) Marriott, Jr., CEO of the Marriott Corporation. "We believe it is absolutely essential to know the markets we serve and what our guests want from us."[1]

As an example, Marriott Hotels asked 27,000 frequent travelers (their target population) which hotel services they ranked most important.

The hotel service most frequently ranked No. 1 was "express check-in."

An Airline Customer Satisfaction Study conducted by J. D. Power and Associates showed that "on-time performance" was 22% of what determined passenger satisfaction. No other single element was judged higher than 15%.[2] Without knowing such priorities, management can only use guesswork, intuition, and trial and error to determine how to best allocate resources to achieve customer satisfaction.

Which of your services do your best patients rank most important? How should you best allocate your resources to boost patient satisfaction, referrals, and practice growth?

This chapter explains numerous ways to obtain that information.

130 Ask a simple question

An outpatient survey from the Williamsport Hospital in Williamsport, PA, asks, "Have you used the Williamsport Hospital Services before? If yes, has the quality of the services improved, remained the same, or declined?"

The first principle in the quest for quality is recognition that quality is what the *patient* perceives it to be, not what you or I say it is (or what it *should* be).

REALITY CHECK

How would your returning patients answer such a survey?

131 Learn patients' preferences

Considering a change in your office hours, perhaps early morning or extended office hours? Rather than impose hours that may work better for *you* than for your patients, *ask them*.

FROM THE SUCCESS FILES

The following is a patient survey from the periodontal office of Richard Roth, D.M.D., J. J. Boscarino, D.M.D., and Kevin Loshak, D.D.S., in Westbury, NY.

Patient Survey
Please assist us in serving you better.
1) Would early morning appointments (between 7 a.m. and 8 a.m.) make coming
    to our office more convenient for you?
2) Are there any of our staff members who should have special acknowledgment?
    Who _____
    Why _____
3) Are there any ways we could improve our service to you?

Your receptionist can give such a survey to patients when they arrive for their appointments, and, because it is short, it most likely can be completed before they leave the office. This will ensure a higher return than a mailed questionnaire.

Another Consideration.   Because of the importance of extended hours, consider distributing such a survey only to your "best patients" (i.e., those whom you would like to see more of in your practice). Reason: There is a good chance their preference for office hours will be representative of non-patients like them.

FROM THE SUCCESS FILES

A Connecticut practitioner starts at 6:00 a.m. to be available to the employees of a local plant who, at that hour, have completed their *late shift* and are headed home. They prefer doing that to making appointments on Saturday.

An Oklahoma practitioner has hours from *4:00 a.m. to 10:00 a.m.* to cater to oil field workers.

Important: "Early morning" or "evening appointments" may mean different things to different people. Be sure to specify in patient surveys the exact times you're considering for extended hours, as well as the days of the week (e.g., Monday, Wednesday, and Friday, starting at 7:00 a.m.).

The second question in the survey pertaining to "staff members who should have special acknowledgment" is indeed "fishing for compliments" (that might otherwise never be expressed). Such feedback provides recognition and reinforcement for those who have earned it and lets everyone know what patients like and appreciate.

132 Anticipate monitoring by managed-care organizations

If your practice is participating in managed care, make sure it earns high marks for patient satisfaction.

Health care organizations are operating in an extremely competitive environment, and patient satisfaction has become key to gaining and maintaining market share. Among the reasons are the following:

- Member dissatisfaction has been shown to be the leading reason for voluntary disenrollment from a plan.
- At a time when many large employers are limiting the number of health plans they offer employees, member dissatisfaction has increasingly become a reason for employers to drop a plan.

Conversely, *satisfied* employees are more likely to

- Re-enroll in a plan
- Pay more to be in a plan
- Request their employer to retain the plan, and
- Encourage others to join their plan.

As a result, managed-care organizations are increasingly using patient satisfaction data when recruiting optometrists and later when deciding whether to deselect or continue working with them.

REALITY CHECK

"With most managed care plans asking enrollees to rate doctors and practices, doctors are well-advised to do some polling of their own," says obstetrician-gynecologist Paul Bluestein, a health maintenance organization medical director who provided the following model survey[3]:

Dear Patient,

We want you to be happy as well as healthy. In order to achieve that goal, we need to know how you and the other women we serve view our practice. We also are interested in learning what changes, if any, you would recommend. We'd be grateful if you would take a minute to complete this brief survey. Your anonymous answers will be very valuable to our ongoing effort to provide friendly, convenient, high-quality care.

Thank you,

	YES	**NO**
Were you greeted promptly and courteously when you arrived?		
Were our billing and insurance policies made clear to you?		
Did you have to wait too long in the reception area before being brought to the examining room?		
Did you have to wait too long in the examining room before the doctor saw you?		
Did the doctor take enough time to listen to everything you had to say and ask?		
Did the doctor thoroughly explain his or her findings and clearly explain instructions for follow-up care?		
Have you had any problems reaching the office after hours or on weekends?		
If a friend were looking for an obstetrician-gynecologist, would you recommend our practice to her?		

If you answered NO to any of the preceding questions, please briefly explain the reasons for your answer(s).

On a scale of 1–5, with 5 signifying the highest degree of satisfaction and 1 the lowest, how would you rate your satisfaction with the following aspects of our practice?

The office	1	2	3	4	5
Our billing and insurance policies	1	2	3	4	5
Our scheduling and punctuality with appointments	1	2	3	4	5
The attention and care you received from our doctors	1	2	3	4	5
Your ability to reach us easily by phone	1	2	3	4	5

Which physician did you see at this visit? Dr. _____

If you could change one thing about our practice, what would it be and how would you change it?

Thank you. Please return this form to the receptionist.

133 Use focus groups

Long used in qualitative market research about consumer products, focus groups are beginning to be used by optometrists to view their practices through the eyes of patients.

A typical focus group consists of eight to ten invited patients who meet for one to 1.0–1.5 hours, usually in the evening, to talk specifically about the practice. The ideal participants are astute, verbal, and willing to speak up about the practice. The preferred setting is a small conference room in a hotel or private room in a restaurant. Light refreshments, such as coffee and cake or fruit and cheese, are typically served.

Many patients are pleased to participate without compensation. Others are more interested if an incentive is offered, such as a credit against future services or purchases.

The ideal person to conduct the session is a professional focus group facilitator who, by definition, is neutral about the practice and more likely to make the participants comfortable enough to express their true feelings, for better or for worse. To locate such a facilitator, contact the school of business at a local college. A professor or perhaps a graduate student may be available. Or, look in the Yellow Pages under "marketing" or "marketing research."

The facilitator should have strong interpersonal skills and be able to start the discussion and then listen without interrupting or getting defensive. He or she should also be strong enough to manage the direction of the discussion while making sure that low-key individuals are not overwhelmed by more outspoken participants.

The following types of questions can be used to start the discussion:

- In your experience with the practice, what have you liked? (It is best to start with a question that everyone will find easy to answer.)
- What if anything, have you disliked? (Participants may at first be hesitant to answer. Be patient: Someone will speak up, and then others will follow.)
- What are some of your "pet peeves" about the office?

- Why did you choose this practice above all others? (See Secret No. 136 for a discussion of the singular importance of this question.)
- Can you think of specific situations that you wish the staff had handled differently?
- Have there been situations that you wish the doctor had handled differently?
- How do you feel about the office environment? Could it be improved in any way?
- How about the office hours? Appointment scheduling?

TARGET POPULATIONS

Do you want more children in your practice? Older patients? Thirty-five- to 50-year-old career people? Computer users? Athletes? Candidates for refractive surgery? Other target populations? Consider focus groups consisting of patients from each of these constituencies: Each will have his or her own point of view and likes and dislikes.

Suggestion.   You'll get better results if the group is homogeneous in terms of education and socioeconomic status. People will be more at ease with each other and more willing to participate in the discussion.

REALITY CHECK

Charles R. Atwood, M.D., a pediatrician in Crowley, LA, says about focus groups, "No matter how much you invite honesty, some people just won't tell you things they're afraid you don't want to hear. So, at the end of each focus group, I pass out index cards and ask patients to write any comments, opinions or criticisms they haven't already expressed—things they'd rather suggest anonymously. Over the years, I've received some doozies."[4]

---

134   Follow up on defections

The average practice loses 10–30% of patients each year. Unfortunately, many of those who defect just quietly leave, never stating their reasons for doing so.

On those occasions, when a patient announces his or her departure by chance, or when you or a staff member learns of it, consider sending the following letter:

Dear [patient's name],
I am sorry to learn from [employee's name] that you've decided to leave our practice. If we have failed to meet your needs or expectations in any way, we'd like to know about it, make amends if possible, and have another chance.
In any event, if we can be of service to you at any time in the future, please don't hesitate to call us.
Sincerely,

This letter leaves the "door open" in case patients find the quality of care and service they receive elsewhere to be unsatisfactory.

Failure to meet expectations is the most common cause of patient dissatisfaction. In many cases, it can be traced back to a badly managed "moment of truth" (see Chapter 6). An apology may be all that's needed. If so, this simple and sincere letter may convince the patient that you are truly sorry and have earned another chance—it's worth a try.

If such a letter could retrieve only one or two patients who made the decision to leave your practice, it would be well worth your efforts.

135 Create an advisory board

To help in long-range planning, many practitioners create advisory boards. Typically, these consist of an accountant, a financial planner, a management consultant, an ophthalmic distributor, and/or other business and professional people who add their knowledge, insights, and perspectives to the management of these practices.

FROM THE SUCCESS FILES

Robert Frazer, Jr., D.D.S., Austin, TX, periodically arranges a nice dinner for a panel of 20 top referring *patients* (called the Select Client Group) who serve as an advisory board to the practice.

In addition to the types of questions asked of a focus group, he also gauges the group's reaction to proposed changes in the practice. A recent topic was the consideration of a separate fee to offset the mounting costs of infection control. The board vetoed the idea.

"In addition," says Dr. Frazer, "we learned that patients do not like calling the office and having the answering service pretend they are part of the office staff. As a result, we now have our answering service identify themselves as the answering service. We learned our patients like to read *Audubon* magazine and have since subscribed to it. And, we learned patients missed the newsletter we had previously written and discontinued; so we reinstituted the publication."

136 Learn why patients choose your office

Many optometrists do not really know why patients have chosen their practice above all others in the community. They can guess and perhaps *hope* that it is for the reasons they would like, but very few actually know for sure.

Without knowing the actual reasons why patients have chosen your practice, the long-range planning for your practice is left to guesswork, trial-and-error, and intuition—all of which may miss the mark. For example, a Brooklyn, NY, optometrist moved his practice a few miles away, believing his patients would surely follow him. As it turned out, large numbers of them *didn't*.

FROM THE SUCCESS FILES

Jack Runninger, O.D., Rome, GA, a former editor of *Optometric Management* and a wise and witty man from whom I've learned a great deal, recounts the story of a lady patient who asked him, "Do you know why I drive 70 miles to come to you for an eye exam? It's inconvenient, and I pass the offices of many good eye doctors on the way," she continued, "yet, I keep coming back to you."

"No, please tell me," he responded, as he (in his words) "pleasurably anticipated the glowing compliments I was about to receive about my skills, charm, and good looks. My ego was soon shattered," he says, "when she replied 'It's because the ladies in your office are so pleasant and always seem happy to see me. That doesn't happen in most doctors' offices!'"[5]

Samuel C. Oliphant, O.D., F.A.A.O., Oklahoma City, OK, focuses primarily on pediatric and contact lens patients and reports, "When we ask new patients why they chose our office they often say, 'I wanted to see a specialist.' We don't ever use the word *specialist* when describing ourselves, but we like the fact that patients perceive us as a specialty practice."[6]

---

137 Learn why your patients *do not* choose your office

Deepak Gupta, O.D., Stamford, CT, candidly admits that he was losing 31% of his contact lens prescriptions and 45% of his spectacle prescriptions to outside sources.

"When I received phone calls from discount chains requesting a verification of a patient's prescription," he says, "I'd call that patient and ask her why she chose not to get her prescription filled at the office. The two main reasons were convenience (patients didn't want to come back to pick up their lenses) and cost.

"The two biggest ways I've found to increase patient retention in contact lens orders," Dr. Gupta says, "are directly shipping to the patient and offering discounted prices for a year's supply of lenses."

The spectacle prescriptions were traced the same way. "I called the 45% of patients who didn't purchase their spectacles at our office and asked them their reasons. Among the main reasons were cost (45%), lack of 1-hour service (35%), and frame selection (15%).

"After remedying these situations," Dr. Gupta says, "I saw contact lens purchases increase from 69% to 85% in one month, and spectacle retention rate go from 50% to 75%. These increases resulted in a year-end $15,000 net profit for the practice."[7]

Leonard J. Press, O.D., F.A.A.O., Fair Lawn, NJ, has used a written patient care survey to monitor patient satisfaction. "Please explain why you did not select eyewear in this office" was one of the questions. The most common explanation? The *perception* that it would be too expensive. It, too, was a situation that was easily remedied.

Feedback, says Ken Blanchard, author of *The One Minute Manager* (Berkley Books, 1983), is the breakfast of champions.

138 Schedule a "no-holds-barred" staff meeting

A low-cost way to undertake marketing research and identify your practice's strengths and weaknesses is to *ask your staff*. Staff members frequently hear patients' comments about the practice but may not share such information. One reason for this is because the optometrists with whom they work never ask.

To tap into this resource, distribute a list of questions to your staff. Then, schedule a "no-holds-barred" meeting to discuss their responses. Sample questions might include the following:

- How would you describe the practice to an outsider?
- What compliments about the practice do you hear most often?
- What complaints do you hear?
- Where, when, and why do misunderstandings with patients most frequently occur? What are your recommendations?
- What changes will improve patient satisfaction?
- What is it about the practice that gives you the greatest pride?

Staff members tend to be more objective about a practice than doctors are. They also view patients from a different perspective and see and hear things that doctors don't. Listen to their ideas and insights: They may open your eyes to opportunities for improved patient satisfaction and practice growth.

139 Conduct post-appointment telephone interviews

This type of follow-up marketing research is done by telephone with 10 or 15 patients representing a cross section of your practice, 2–3 days after their appointments. The interviews are most often done by an office manager and/or staff members on a rotating basis. The premise is to sensitize everyone to the importance of *patient satisfaction.*

To expedite the interviews, have a staff member make advance arrangements with preselected patients at the conclusion of their appointments. For example,

"Mrs. Carlson, we plan to call a few of the patients seen this week to ask about their experiences while being in our office. We'd very much like your opinion on this topic. Would you be willing to be interviewed for just a few minutes later this week, at any time that's convenient to you?"

Most patients are agreeable, if not flattered, to be interviewed. The following are some suggested questions to ask such patients:

- How did everything go during your appointment?
- Were all of your questions answered?
- Was there anything, big or small, that bothered you in any way?
- Is there anything we could have done to make your visit a more positive experience?
- If a friend were looking for an optometrist, would you be comfortable in recommending our practice?

TESTED TIP

As in any interview, the more you draw the person out, the more you learn. Phrases such as "that's interesting" and "tell me more about that" let patients know the interviewer is truly interested in what they have to say.

An alternative to the post-appointment telephone interview is simply to have the receptionist ask patients as they are paying the bill at the conclusion of the visit, "How did everything go today?" In asking such a question, it is important to hold eye contact with the patient and look genuinely interested. Otherwise, the patient may not attach any importance to the question and simply say "fine."

Regardless of what you hear—brickbats or bouquets—the feedback you obtain from such interviews will help you identify hidden "blind spots" about your practice.

140 Success stories

"'Success Stories are patients' and parents' reports of gains achieved through vision therapy," says Martin B. Birnbaum, O.D., New Hyde

Park, NY. "They serve several purposes: They help the patient and parent recognize and be more aware of the behavioral changes that have occurred and the degree to which their goals have been achieved. When a patient's therapy is concluded, inclusion of the Success Story with a report to the referring professional provides the referring professional with a statement of the gains achieved, in the patient's own words. It also fosters a greater confidence in vision therapy as a treatment modality and encourages increased referrals. Most importantly, Success Stories also reveal the tremendous impact that vision therapy has on people's lives."

FROM THE SUCCESS FILES

The survey used in Dr. Birnbaum's office is as follows:

Please Share Your Success with Others

We have enjoyed treating you and are pleased that substantial improvement in visual function has been achieved. Patients often note that improved visual function brings changes in school performance, work performance, sports, and even in attitude and personality. We would appreciate you describing below any changes you have observed as a result of vision therapy. We'd also appreciate your permission to share this with others who may have little knowledge of vision therapy.

Date_____ Name_____
Permission to share?   Yes   No
Would you recommend vision therapy to others?   Yes   No

"What comes through in reading the Success Stories that patients write," says Dr. Birnbaum, "is not only the elimination of asthenopia, diplopia, loss of place when reading, and other symptoms of functional vision disorder, but rather, improved school achievement, improved ability to sustain attention and improved sports performance. In addition, children whose vision problems are at the root of their school difficulty, often come to believe that they are indeed stupid or lazy. Following remediation of vision dysfunctions, they frequently report heightened self-esteem as a consequence of improved life achievement. These reports have, in turn, heightened my awareness of the degree to which vision disorders that interfere with learning and achievement cause poor self-image, poor self-esteem, and attendant psychological problems."

"The use of Success Stories," says Dr. Birnbaum, "has contributed significantly to both my practice development and to my professional growth."[8]

141 Audit yourself

Question: After an exam, what percentage of your recommendations for vision therapy, contact lenses, premium lens options, and the like are *accepted* by patients? If it's not as high as you would like, one reason may have to do with *how* you say *what* you say to patients.

REALITY CHECK

You probably haven't had your communication skills critiqued in a long time, if ever. And, may the truth be known, no one is likely to tell you about your shortcomings as a communicator. The easiest, most practical way to learn how you come across to others is to audit yourself by *tape recording* your interactions with patients. You may be highly pleased with what you hear—*or* you may be taken aback. Either way, it is worth a listen.

Among the *communication blunders* you may unintentionally be making are the following:

Too Technical. Doctors often explain their findings and recommendations in language that patients don't understand. Rather than admit it and look foolish, many patients just nod their heads and pretend to understand.

REALITY CHECK

Patients can't accept what they don't understand.

Too Rushed. When explaining glaucoma, for example, and the importance of medication and follow-up exams for the five-hundredth time (especially if you are time pressured), it is easy to fall into the trap of speaking so fast that patients cannot follow. Again, some pretend to understand when, in fact, they don't. The predictable result? Lack of compliance.

Talking Too Much. Another well-intentioned habit that no one is ever going to tell you about is the tendency to talk too much, telling patients *more* than they want to know or *need to know*. Listen to yourself. You may start to squirm as you hear yourself going on and on and on and on and on . . . .

High Pressure. It's natural to want patients to accept your recommendations, but continuing to "sell" after patients say "no" or "I'd like to think about it" may come across as "pushy." What you say may be well intentioned, but if it is *perceived* as "high-pressure" it undermines trust and make patients uncomfortable.

REALITY CHECK

Today's more savvy, discerning, and demanding patient has less patience than ever for the "hard sell" and more opportunity to obtain eye care and eyewear elsewhere.

The issue is not how technical, rushed, talkative, or high-pressure you *are*, but rather how technical, rushed, talkative, or high-pressure you're *perceived* to be.

Audit yourself to learn if you're as good a communicator as you think you are.

HARD-LEARNED LESSON

"In order to learn from mistakes, you first have to recognize you are making mistakes."[9]

CAVEAT

The permissibility of taping a conversation without a patient's knowledge and consent varies from state to state. Check with your attorney to learn what obligations, if any, you have in this regard.

142   Mystery shopping

In the context of professional practice, "mystery shoppers" are really *mystery patients*, anonymous evaluators who provide insights into how well everyone in the practice, from receptionist to doctor, is serving patients.

Here is how one practice evaluated itself with mystery shopping.

Suzanne Bruno, ophthalmic administrator of Horizon Eye Care, Margate, NJ, recruited mystery patients to visit their five offices and surgery center. All were members of a local civic association, but only she knew who they were. The practice made a charitable donation to the civic group and provided complimentary exams and 50% discounts on eyewear to all participants.

A few of the mystery shoppers, including two who needed cataract surgery, were already patients in the practice. The rest were new patients, most of whom stayed with the practice. They paid for their visits and were reimbursed on the receipts. It took a huge effort on Ms. Bruno's part to develop the lengthy questionnaire she distributed to the mystery shoppers, communicate secretly with these patients, process all their refunds, and compile evaluations, but the feedback has been invaluable.

For example, being "child friendly" was a practice goal, so some of the volunteers were asked to bring their children in for exams. "We discovered," Ms. Bruno says, "that our staff and our doctors were good with children but our office wasn't. That's one thing we changed as a direct result of the program. All our offices now have toy boxes with books, toys, and even video games for older children."[10]

SAMPLE MYSTERY PATIENT QUESTIONS

Was the phone answered on three rings?
How long did you have to wait for an appointment?
Were you greeted promptly when you entered the office?
How long did you wait before being taken into a room for the pre-exam?
Was the facility clean?
Were exam procedures explained clearly?
Were you given an opportunity to ask the doctor questions?
Were your glasses/contact lenses ready when promised?

HARD-LEARNED LESSON

Trying to achieve a high-performance optometric practice without *feedback* is like trying to learn target shooting with a blindfold—it can't be done.

143 Survey your referrers

Once your relationship with professional colleagues is established and referrals start coming in, you will want to learn whether you and your staff are meeting their expectations. Do you see referred patients quickly enough? Do you provide the full range of services they seek? Are your reports sent promptly? Do they have enough information? Perhaps too much? Is your office staff friendly and helpful to the referring doctor and their patients?

To obtain such information, consider sending a short, written survey to your referrers, including those who may only send you an occasional referral. Make the questions easy to answer with a "yes" or "no" (or with a ranking from 1 [poor] to 5 [excellent]) and leave space for additional comments.

FROM THE SUCCESS FILES

Anthony A. Sirianni, D.D.S., John P. Graziano, D.D.S., Martin P. Epstein, D.D.S., and Robert W. Weeman, D.D.S., who maintain orthodontic practices in Brooklyn and Staten Island, NY, include, among others, the following three questions in their surveys of referring dentists:

- Do you prefer phone calls_____ a.m.?_____p.m.?_____ after hours? No special time_____?
- Would you like your staff to come to our office for a "lunch and learn" discussion of basic orthodontic diagnosis and treatment planning, temporomandibular joint dysfunction, orthognathic surgery? Yes_____ No_____ Future_____
- Do you have any comments or suggestions for developing a better relationship between our offices?_____

REALITY CHECK

Don't be surprised if referring physicians have widely different needs, interests, and priorities. The more that you and your staff can accommodate their individual preferences, the more effective your relationships will be.

Ralph Waldo Emerson observed, "The field cannot be seen from within the field." This sampling of marketing research techniques enables you to get that all-important *outside view* of your practice— through the eyes of patients, mystery patients, staff members, and referral sources.

Notes

1. Back to School. *Incentive*, March 1993, 25.
2. Krauss P. *The Book of Management Wisdom*. New York: John Wiley & Sons Inc., 2000.
3. Bluestein P. Getting a Handle on Patient Satisfaction. *OBG Management*, October 1995, 49.
4. Atwood CR. Give These Little Extras and Watch Your Practice Grow. *Medical Economics*, March 2, 1992, 133–143.
5. Runninger J. Two Ears, One Mouth. *Optometric Management*, December 1999, 10.
6. Strategies to Grow Your Contact Lens Practice. Healthy Patients, Healthy Practices. Supplement to *Optometric Management*, July 2001, 3S–6S.
7. Gupta D. Turning Your Revenue Around. *Optometric Management*, September 2001, 77–78,81–82.
8. Birnbaum MH. Success Stories. *Journal of Behavioral Optometry*, Volume 9, Number 3, 1998, 67–69,77.
9. Wall Street Journal editorial, January 9, 1982.
10. Beiting J. Taking the Mystery Out of Patient Satisfaction. *Quirk's Marketing Research Review*, January 2001, 16,48–49.

9

Get the Right People on Board

The hiring of employees is the single most important management task you do. These important members of the vision care team greatly influence patient satisfaction, as well as the productivity and profitability of your practice. They also shape the "personality" and reputation of your practice, not only among patients, but just as important, among physicians and other referral sources.

The first step: Get the right people on board.

144 Know what you are looking for

Identify the skills, experience, values, and personality traits of the person you are looking for: It will simplify the search.

That may not be as easy as it first seems, however. At the workshops I conduct on personnel management, I ask optometrists and office managers to describe, for example, the ideal receptionist. The resulting profiles vary from one practice to another and sometimes from one individual to another in the same practice.

NEXT STEP

The following list of character traits are those most frequently listed by workshop participants. Add others of your own choosing, then select the five or so traits you consider most important. Doing so greatly simplifies the task of finding the person you seek.

ambitious	good listener	resourceful
cheerful	hard working	respectful
common sense	honest	responsible
conscientious	imaginative	self-confident
courteous	independent	self-motivated
creative	intelligent	sense of humor
curious	kind	sensitive
detail oriented	likable	sincere
diplomatic	likes challenge	team player
eager to learn	loyal	tenacious
empathetic	patient	thorough
energetic	perceptive	tolerance for contact
enthusiastic	persistent	(see Secret No. 145)
flexible	personable	warm
focused	polite	works well under
friendly	productive	pressure
goal oriented	punctual	

145 High tolerance for contact

Anyone dealing with the public, day after day, engages in what sociologist Arlie Hochschild calls "emotional labor." It refers to the kind of work where "feelings" such as cheerfulness, warmth, and sympathetic concern are an important part of job performance. Optometrists and their staffs are prime examples. Having to display such emotions with patients, day after day, whether or not you feel like it, is taxing—especially in a high-volume practice.

Above all, such repetitive encounters require what's called a *high tolerance for contact*. Those who lack it can become moody, irritable, and perhaps short-tempered with patients. In time, they may burn out from the demands of emotional labor.

Reality Check

If you are in practice and lack a high tolerance for contact, the best thing you can do is to surround yourself with people who have it in abundance.

146 What others look for

"What's the most important trait you look for in a new employee— beyond skills and experience?" is a question I have asked countless doctors. The answer given by Dr. Steven Garner, A.B.V.P., owner and chief of staff of Safari Animal Care Centers in League City, TX, and his wife and hospital administrator, Cheryl B. Garner, was *"Nice. We can train people to do almost anything,"* they say, *"but we can't make them nice."*

Nancy G. Torgerson, O.D., F.C.O.V.D., Lynnwood, WA, whose practice is limited to vision therapy, looks for employees who have "enthusiasm, empathy, and a love of learning."

The EuroDisney Theme Park (outside Paris, France) is a highly acclaimed, service-driven organization. What traits do they look for when hiring critically important personnel who deal with a demanding public?

The following is an excerpt from a help-wanted ad for EuroDisney: "We need strong team players with

* Exceptional people skills
* Constant smiles
* Never-say-no attitudes
* Friendly, helpful, courteous"

Charles Blair, D.D.S., a dentist and management consultant in Charlotte, NC, searches for employees with the following traits, beginning with what he considers the most important:

1. Loyalty
2. Stability

3. Enthusiasm
4. Judgment
5. Intelligence
6. Technical ability

Surprised that the top-ranked characteristics are so subjective? "Creating a conscientious, effective and efficient team," says Dr. Blair, "depends more on those personality traits than on IQ, computer literacy, or credentials."

Jeff Bezos, Amazon.com's founder and CEO, wants to know if job applicants can "bring something extra to the company—some *zing*—some *zip*—some *lift*. Many people," he says, "have unique skills, interests, and perspectives that enrich the work environment for all of us."[1]

ACTION STEP

Circulate the list of character traits to all staff members and ask each person to check the five traits he or she considers most important in a co-worker. Discuss the results at a staff meeting and reach a consensus. Doing so establishes standards for new as well as current staff members.

147 Creatively recruit new employees

Finding the right people for your practice who are loyal, hard working, nice, eager to learn, and able to leap tall buildings is not easy, especially in a tight job market. If the usual recruiting channels are not producing qualified candidates, consider offering a recruiting bonus of $300–$500 to any staff member who recommends an individual who, after a 90-day probationary period, is subsequently hired. If an employee you respect likes someone well enough to recommend him or her, the odds are better than average that the new person will fit in with your staff.

At the outset, make it clear that the same high standards and selection process will be used to evaluate job applicants recommended by staff members. Stating this policy up front helps avoid any obligation you may feel to hire someone you do not consider the best choice for your practice.

REALITY CHECK

A recent survey by Referral Networks, a New York City–based company, offers some insights into what motivates employees to make referrals. The news is good: Monetary incentives are not what drive the process. Forty-two percent of the 2,300 employees surveyed said they referred because they wanted to help a friend find a good job. Twenty-four percent said they wanted to help the company. Another 24% said they were motivated by a reward.[2]

TESTED TIP

If one of your *patients* has all the traits you are looking for in an employee, consider recruiting him or her. You might ask, "I'd love to have someone with your personality working here. Do you know of anyone?" The person may be interested in the job or know someone who might be. I know of many optometric staff members who were hired exactly this way.

148   Use part-time employees

If you answer "yes" to one or more of the following questions, your practice may benefit from hiring *part-time employees*.

- Have you had difficulty finding qualified, full-time office personnel?
- Does your practice have peaks and valleys of activity?
- Does your staff lack the time to implement ideas that would generate practice growth?
- Do your employees have child or elder care obligations that impinge on their work schedule?
- Has burnout become a problem for any of your employees?
- Has employee turnover been a problem in your practice?

In many areas of the country, part-time employees are the fastest growing segment of the labor force. Among the many benefits of hiring them are the following:

- Greatly increases the pool of applicants, including those who may have left the profession to start a family and now want to return to work on a part-time basis.
- Provides a tremendous recruitment edge when other practices offer the same compensation but no part-time option.
- Helps smooth the peaks and valleys of workflow and improve patient service at the busiest times.
- Improves productivity and morale. Because of a reduced workweek, part-time employees bring increased energy to the job. They are also able to better focus on their work and usually miss fewer days.
- Retains older employees who have valuable skills and experience. Surveys indicate many members of this age group would extend their working life *if* they could work part time, rather than choose between full-time work and retirement. For example, Dr. Stuart Gindoff (see "From the Success Files" section that follows) has retained two valuable employees who, after many years of employment, requested part-time status and were granted it.
- Reduces labor costs during slow times when full-time employees are not needed. Also, as a general rule, employers are not required under current law to provide fringe benefits for employees who work fewer than 1,000 hours per year. Check your state's requirements.

ONE CAVEAT

Part-time employees may feel like outsiders or "second-class" citizens. To foster a connection, schedule staff meetings at times so they can attend, keep them informed about policy and protocol changes, and provide frequent performance feedback.

FROM THE SUCCESS FILES

Stuart Gindoff, O.D., M.B.A., F.A.A.O., managing partner of the Eye Center South in Sarasota, FL, reports, "We have four part-time employees and are extremely satisfied with the arrangement. One reason: the saving in overhead costs. For example, our part-time employees realize they won't be paid sick time, do not accumulate vacation time, and won't be paid when the office is closed for a holiday (unless it is a regularly scheduled workday). It's also understood their status does not require a contribution on our part to a retirement fund.

"Another major advantage," Dr. Gindoff adds, "is that we're able to have more than one employee trained to do a specific job. Should illness or unexpected absences occur, 'substitutes' can be called."

"Is *consistency* a problem?" I asked.

"For the most part, it's not been a problem," he replied. "However, if there's a visible difference between two part-timers doing the same job, then it's the supervisor's (or doctor's) responsibility to straighten things out.

"We've successfully used part-time personnel for the last several years," Dr. Gindoff says. "If we didn't have such a trained ophthalmic labor shortage in our area, we'd hire even more."

149   Offer family-friendly perks

Not long ago, a good salary and a basic benefits package were enough to entice skilled job applicants to join a practice, and once on board, to remain there. In a strong economy, however, applicants have the upper hand in terms of which jobs they accept and how long they stay—with the option of "job hopping" if they're dissatisfied. The average American worker holds 9.2 jobs from age 18–34 years, according to the U.S. Labor Department's Bureau of Labor Statistics.

If you are experiencing a shortage of skilled job applicants and/or high employee turnover, consider adding to your package of basic benefits some of the following family-friendly perks now being offered by an increasing number of employers:

- Flextime (flexible work hours)
- Compressed workweek (work longer days in exchange for a shorter week)
- Job sharing (e.g., divide one full-time job into two part-time jobs)
- Telecommuting opportunities (work at home with computer, fax, and modem)
- Paid "personal days" to be used for any purpose
- Paid maternity-paternity leave

- On-site child care (e.g., provided by a senior citizen)
- Tuition-paid continuing education
- On-site fitness equipment (e.g., treadmill)
- Staff lounge (e.g., with microwave, refrigerator)
- Special areas, other than bathrooms, where working moms can breast-feed their babies. (Studies cite a decreased rate of absenteeism where this is allowed.)

Family-friendly perks like many of those previously mentioned are more effective at retaining valuable employees than cash incentives, according to 352 human resource executives surveyed by the American Management Association.

REALITY CHECK

"It would be nice to offer your employees a world of benefits," says Pamela Miller, O.D., J.D., Highland, CA. "Unfortunately, that's not realistic. So find out what they need most."[3]

ACTION STEP

Conduct one-on-one interviews with employees to learn which "perks" of those you're willing to offer are of greatest interest.

Family-friendly perks can ease the conflicts many employees have between home and work, reduce turnover, and enhance on-the-job performance. They can also be highly appealing to prospective employees in a tight labor market. Include them in classified ads.

150 Avoid costly hiring mistakes

Have you ever hired someone who sounded great in the interview, and then fell short on the job? What went wrong?

Job seekers have become increasingly savvy and are better prepared for job interviews than ever before. There are countless books and Internet sites to help them look good on a job interview and get the job they want. In addition, because of the litigious times in which we live, even reference checks may fail to give you the whole story about a job applicant.

I have asked countless personnel managers in a wide range of businesses and professions what interview questions they've found most helpful in judging job applicants: The following is a sampling. What is good about these questions is that job applicants have no way of knowing the needs of your practice or exactly what *you are* looking for. Their best choice is to be honest and straightforward.

- What are you looking for in your next job that is missing from your present one?
- Do you prefer to work alone or with others?
- What about your work do you find most challenging?
- What aspects of your last job did you like best? Least?
- What job-related situations have you found most stressful?
- What have you found most effective in dealing with such stress?
- What do you consider your greatest strengths? Don't be modest.
- In which of your jobs did you learn the most?
- Tell me about the best boss you ever had. What about the worst?
- (If the position involves fee discussions or collections) How do you feel about asking people for money? (Surprisingly, some job applicants in an off-guard moment admit they don't like these tasks.)
- Have you ever seen an optometric assistant/receptionist/technician (depending on the position for which you are hiring) show especially poor judgment? If so, tell me about it.

TESTED TIP

For best results, probe for further information with such follow-up requests as "please explain" or "that's interesting, tell me more."

151 Uncover a job applicant's "inner traits"

After considering job skills and experience, many optometrists tend to appraise job applicants according to appearance, communication skills, and sociability or personality. Although these are important traits for an optometric office, they're not enough.

Far more important than personality and the like are a person's *inner traits*: intelligence, inner drive, attitude toward work, and the ability to get along with others, to name a few. These factors determine whether a person with the right job skills and experience is right for your practice.

Here are more tested interview questions to help elicit information about these inner traits:

- In your last job, what did you do that you are most proud of?
- In your last job, when you finished your work ahead of schedule, what did you usually do?
- Do you like someone who gives you a lot of responsibility or someone who provides a lot of supervision?
- Have you learned any new skills or explored some new field of interest, even a hobby, since leaving school?

As a final question, consider asking a job applicant "Is there anything you'd like to discuss that we haven't talked about?" See if the person asks about job content, your expectations, why the last person left, or other related questions that may provide clues to the person's "inner traits."

Long pauses or no answers to such questions can be highly revealing.

152 Ask behavior-based questions

Behavior-based questions require job applicants to reveal specific information about how they handled particular situations in the past. The purpose is to predict a person's *future performance* based on his or her *past job experience*. The following are some examples of questions:

- In your previous job(s), were you ever asked to stay late on a day when you had other plans? What did you do and how did you feel about it?

- Describe a time when you encountered obstacles in your last job while you were in pursuit of a goal. What happened?
- Describe a situation that occurred in your last job that required great patience on your part. How did you deal with it?
- Have you ever had to deal with an irate patient (customer, client)? What happened?
- Have you ever had to deal with co-workers who did not cooperate or contribute a fair share of the work? What did you do in those situations?

REALITY CHECK

As revealing as the replies to such questions might be in evaluating a job applicant, not all candidates are going to be comfortable in answering them. Use such questions sparingly and move on to other matters as the situation warrants.

153 Hire "likable" people

Some staff members are extremely personable and instantly likable; others are less so. And oh, what a difference it makes in the rhythm of the office, the image of the practice, patient satisfaction, and everyone's "mood" at the end of the day.

A likable personality is a priceless asset (some say "necessity") in any service occupation, optometry included. It is frequently underestimated by management, however, or completely overlooked during the hiring process.

What is a "likable personality?" Bobbie Gee, former image and appearance coordinator for Disneyland, says likable people

- Smile easily
- Have a good sense of humor
- Are great listeners
- Know common-sense etiquette and use it
- Compliment easily and often
- Are self-confident

- Engage you in conversation about yourself
- Can laugh at themselves
- Are approachable[4]

When interviewing job applicants, pay special attention to their personalities. Do they have the aforementioned traits or others you deem important? Ask current employees to judge how likable and friendly they are—it raises everyone's awareness of the "Likable Factor" and its importance to a successful practice.

154   How likable are you?

In his book, *Kids Don't Learn from People They Don't Like*, author/educator David Aspy writes that when students don't like a teacher, they develop a resistance to learning. Students, it seems, do best with teachers they *like*.

Our surveys indicate the same is true in the workplace. When employees like the optometrists and office managers with whom they work, there tends to be less absenteeism and turnover; better morale and motivation; and more teamwork and productivity. They also speak openly about how much they love their jobs.

Take another look at those traits of the "likable personality." Does any of them need a little polishing on your part?

155   Check out the person's "view of the world"

"Nothing better indicates a candidate's confidence than his or her view of the world in general," writes Robert Half, president of the recruiting firm Robert Half International, Inc. "Are they optimistic or pessimistic?" he asks. "Do they view the proverbial glass as half empty or half full? People with a positive viewpoint are infinitely more likely to be happier, more productive, and more efficient. They are easier to motivate, quicker to learn, and adapt to a variety of situations, and in general, have greater potential to become top-notch employees."

When evaluating competing candidates for a job, Half recommends that when all else is equal, chose the person who most wants the job.[5]

FROM THE SUCCESS FILES

In the office of Nancy G. Torgerson, O.D., F.C.O.V.D., Lynnwood, WA, job applicants are invited to observe vision therapy sessions or parent-teacher workshops conducted in her office. Current staff members then note if the applicants are well mannered, if they listen, if they interact well with patients, and if they appear comfortable doing so.

As a follow-up, Dr. Torgerson, her office manager, and her vision therapy administrator take the "finalists" to lunch and then make their decision.

---

156 Hard-learned lessons about hiring

- If a new employee doesn't have the right attitude about work or the right personality for your practice, it's unlikely a written script of what to say to patients or even on-the-job training is going to make a difference.
- "Staff your company," says consultant Ron Zemke, "with people who don't see their jobs as burdens and chores. Look for individuals who get a kick out of serving other people. Look for employees who find customer contact exciting and rewarding—who don't find any aspect of serving others demeaning. They're the ones who will deliver service that will set your business apart."[6]
- Every employee contributes to a patient's impression of your office—for better or for worse.
- Compromising your standards because the pool of job applicants is small and you are desperate is what I call the "buy now, pay later" approach to hiring.
- Beware of the "Halo Effect"—being so dazzled by one quality of a job applicant (e.g., appearance, friendliness, computer skills) that you lose sight of other important job requirements.

- Beware of a history of "job hopping." Three jobs in 5 years may be too many unless the changes show a sensible pattern, say, higher pay or more responsibility.
- Beware of job applicants who reveal confidential information about former employers, practices, or patients. You'll be next.
- Your practice is only as strong as your weakest employee.
- Don't oversell a job by promising more than you can deliver or, conversely, by downplaying the negative aspects of a job. When the facts become known, a new employee either becomes demotivated or quits. Face the facts: *A job is what it is.* One solution: Rethink the position. Can the appealing aspects of the job be broadened? Can less-desirable aspects be traded or possibly divided among other employees, or perhaps outsourced?
- Always ask job applicants, "What am I likely to hear, positive and negative, when I call your references?" The question gives them an opportunity to brag about their previous job strengths and achievements. It also enables them to tell their side of any negative story you might hear (or one they *think* you might hear).
- Allow employees to interview job applicants and to narrow the list down to a few from which you will make the final selection. Or, let your staff have the final approval of someone you tentatively have decided to hire. Employees will get along better with each other and have more team spirit if they have some say in the hiring of new employees, as opposed to your doing it completely on your own.
- Never hire someone whose first question is, "What are the benefits?"
- Never hire someone you can't fire, such as friends and relatives.
- Never hire someone who's not quite right for job with the expectation he or she will change. Dr. L. D. Panky said it best: You can change people, but not very much.
- As certain as you might be that you have found the perfect candidate, resist the temptation to hire somebody on the spot unless you've been unable to fill the job for a long time and delay could jeopardize your chances of hiring the person. In general, though, it is always good to give yourself a day or two to make sure you're not overlooking faults that could later surface. The best approach: Let the candidate know you're interested and ask for a day or two to make the final decision.

Notes

1. Davis B. *Speed Is Life: Street Smart Lessons from the Front Lines of Business*. New York: Currency, 2001.
2. Lachnitt C. Employee Referral. *Workforce*, June 2001, 67–72.
3. Black A. Benefits: Money Well Spent? *Review of Optometry*, June 2001, 37.
4. Gee B. *Creating a Million Dollar Image for Your Business: Smart Strategies for Building an Image That Works*. Berkeley, CA: Pagemill Press, 1996.
5. Half R. *Finding, Hiring, and Keeping the Best Employees*. New York: John Wiley & Sons, 1993.
6. Zemke R. Secrets of "Knock Your Socks Off" Service. *Bottom Line Business*, April 1998.

10

Brass Tacks of Personnel Management

Let's start with a few troubling but obvious facts: Employee turnover is expensive. Finding new talent is challenging. Training new people is time consuming. Retaining employees once they have gained experience and expertise at your expense continues to be difficult. Low levels of employee satisfaction threaten staff morale, patient relations, and practice growth, and, in turn, lead to profit-draining high turnover rates.

On the other hand, high levels of employee satisfaction mean increased motivation and productivity, greater patient satisfaction and referrals (as employees communicate their enthusiasm for your practice, services, and products), lower levels of employee turnover, and higher profitability.

157 High cost of turnover

To calculate your annual employee turnover rate, divide this year's number of employee defections by the total number of staff, then multiply by 100. "If the staff turnover rate exceeds 15% on average over the last 5 years, your practice is considered to have high turnover," says California consultant Judy Capko.[1]

Employee replacement costs are estimated at 25% of annual compensation, including the costs of recruitment, training, and the time a new employee takes to reach his or her maximum efficiency level. Turnover also results in a huge toll on staff morale and patient satisfaction. So, focusing your attention on improving staff retention rates can accomplish much more than just improving your bottom line.

158 Delegation

"If you have a small or average size practice ($350,000 gross) and are amazed at how some optometrists can individually gross $500,000 or $1,000,000 or more," says Jerry Hayes, O.D., Director of Hayes Consulting, "I'll tell you one of their secrets: A lot of the work gets done by their staffs."[2]

In the era of managed care, delegation has become an imperative to operate at peak efficiency. Yet, many optometrists are performing tasks in their practices that could be done just as well, perhaps better, and definitely at less cost, by appropriately trained staff. The tasks are in all areas of the practice: Some are related to management, many are of a clinical nature, and some are just routine chores.

Many doctors of optometry justify their failure to delegate by saying, "If I want it done right, I have to do it myself." Unfortunately, this line of reasoning becomes a self-fulfilling prophecy. Employees cannot learn to do what optometrists insist on doing themselves, so the doctors keep on doing what they have always done.

If you are a do-it-yourself optometrist, there is a lot to be gained if you're willing to loosen the reins a little to allow qualified employees to take on new responsibilities. Delegation frees you to see more patients. Do more of what only you can do: Focus on refractive disorders, binocular vision, and ocular health.

Employees interested in personal growth, job enrichment, and broader responsibilities benefit as well. Their earning potential increases, as well as their pride and job satisfaction.

REALITY CHECK

The real question, as Irvin Borish, O.D., D.O.S., LL.D., D.Sc., the man known as optometry's architect, asked, is, *Do you want to be a data gatherer or data analyzer?*

Do you prefer to do all the tests yourself? Limit yourself to just a few exams per hour? *Or*, delegate as much of a comprehensive eye exam as is legally possible to qualified technicians and instead, limit yourself to evaluating the data, diagnosing problems, designing treatment plans, and conferring with patients?

These are two very different styles of practice, each having different staffing requirements.

159 Hard-learned lessons about delegation

* "Patients perceive more value in our services," says Walter D. West, O.D., F.A.A.O., Brentwood, TN, "when I spend more time talking and educating rather than gathering clinical data."[3]
* "Modern optometry," says Dr. Irvin Borish, "must not only persist in expanding its scope; it must also continue to maintain its precision and dominance in the major areas of its fundamentals. This is made possible by using technicians and the latest automated equipment; by delegating techniques that determine quantitative data and reserving professional time for those which demand qualitative evaluation, concentrated listening to, and understanding of patients' problems; determination of suitable procedures; and diagnosis and analysis of possible solutions."[4]
* Although delegation is a proven way to increase productivity and the job satisfaction of the staff member to whom a higher-level task is delegated, *it's not for everyone*. Some doctors of optometry prefer not to let go of the reins, and some staff members don't want the responsibility of taking them.
* "Intelligent delegation," says Neil B. Gailmard, O.D., M.B.A., F.A.A.O., Munster, IN, "can definitely take your practice to the next level of efficiency and productivity."[5]

REALITY CHECK

Delegation requires a willingness to accept some mistakes along the way. Without risk, there is no growth.

160 Flexible sick-leave policy

What happens when employees are needed at home to care for a sick child, spouse, or other family member? Do they call in "sick" and take the day off? Do they come to work, yet remain distracted by the at-home situation? The answer depends on several factors, one of which is the flexibility of your sick-leave policy.

An employee benefit that is becoming more widely offered extends conventional sick leave to include other times when family members are ill. Called *family sick leave*, it eliminates the need to fake an illness and then lie about it. In the end, it doesn't cost you any more.

Typically, family sick leave is computed at the rate of one-half day for each month worked (after a 90-day probationary period), up to a total of 6 days a year. What about unused sick days? Increasingly, employees are being paid for them. Doing so provides an incentive to get to work for those undecided about making the effort.

An alternative way of dealing with unused sick days is to accumulate them in a "paid-leave bank" up to a maximum 20–30 days per employee. These days can then be used for such emergencies as a major illness or surgery, allowing employees to take the time needed for recuperation without losing pay.

An Alaska practitioner credits 2 hours of vacation time for employees who don't use sick leave during an entire calendar month. A staff member not taking sick leave for 6 months receives an extra day-and-a-half of vacation time.

Keep in mind that flexible personnel policies are helpful in attracting and retaining top-notch employees.

TESTED TIP

When first interviewing job applicants, you can get a sense of their attitude toward sick-day absences by asking such questions as the following:

• What do you think constitutes a good attendance record?
• What do you consider to be good reasons for missing work?

Special Situation: Extended Absence Owing to Illness or Injury. Employees on extended leave owing to illness or injury tend to return to work sooner, says *Personnel Journal*, if employers stay in touch. Ongoing personal contact reassures employees they are valued, have not been forgotten, and are missed on the job. Older workers often fear that they could be replaced by younger people and may need their employer's reassurance even more.[6]

161 Have written job descriptions

Try this experiment: Ask your employees to write a list of their job duties and responsibilities. Ask them to include every last thing they think is expected of them. Explain that you will do the same for each of their jobs. Then, *compare* the lists.

If your office does not have *written* job descriptions, your lists probably will not match those of your employees. That discrepancy, if it exists, can lead to misunderstandings between you and your employees, or even between employees themselves, as to "who does what."

A study by the American Management Association indicates that a shocking seven out of ten employees do not know exactly what is expected of them on the job. The term used to describe this confusion is *role ambiguity*.

To make matters worse, many employers are not sure what their employees are supposed to do, either. They have never summarized, in written form, the required knowledge and skills for each position or the precise duties and responsibilities expected of each employee. As a result, there are only vague guidelines for the hiring and periodic evaluation of employees.

ACTION STEPS

The management tool needed to eliminate such confusion is a *written job description* for each position. To clarify what is expected, include the following:

- *Job Title*:
- *Reports to*: This defines the employee's line of communication regarding office operations, policies, job-related complaints, special privileges, salary reviews, vacations, and related matters.
- *Duties and Responsibilities*: This identifies the individual tasks that each employee is expected to perform. It may also include the frequency with which these tasks are to be performed (e.g., daily, weekly, monthly, as needed). For example: "Each day, before the first patient arrives, make lists of the day's appointments and post one in each exam room, the doctor's private office, and the dispensing area. The list should include appointment times, patients' names, and scheduled services."

The more detail you include, the less chance of confusion and resentment. For example, two common employee gripes are "My job has not turned out to be the way it was described to me when I was hired," and, when asked to do what an employee considers to be a nonroutine task, "I didn't know this was part of my job."

Written job descriptions help to eliminate such misunderstandings.

Note: One clause frequently found in job descriptions is "other duties as needed." This "escape clause," written for management's benefit, is unfair and negates the very purpose of a job description.

- *Required Skills and Knowledge*: For example—the ability to take health histories, do vision screenings, noncontact tonometry, autorefractions, computerized field screenings, blood pressure readings, and fundus photography.

Jobs change as your practice grows; as employees acquire new knowledge, skills, and interests; perhaps as legislation is passed; or as job turnover occurs. For job descriptions to be effective, they need to reflect each position's current requirements. If 2 years have elapsed or more than two people have held the same position since a job description was first written, it's probably obsolete.

HARD-LEARNED LESSON

Involve employees in writing and updating job descriptions. After all, who knows a job better than the person who actually does it?

If you and your employees come up with different lists of duties and responsibilities for any job, negotiate the tasks in question. The point is to reach agreement on what is expected of each employee.

162 Do your employees realize how much they are paid?

Many optometric staff members I have interviewed look at their compensation strictly in terms of *take-home pay*—without considering the substantial *fringe benefits* they also receive. Knowing all the facts makes employees realize how much they are actually paid and often has an immediate and highly positive impact on morale and motivation.

To make employees aware of the total compensation they receive, provide them annually with a *Total Pay Statement* like the following, with their W-2 form. List the dollar value of the many extras your practice offers that otherwise may be overlooked or taken for granted.

Total Pay Statement

This statement is a summary of the various forms of compensation you receive as a staff member of this practice.

Benefit	Value ($)
Gross base salary	
Overtime and bonuses	
Health insurance (for employee and dependents)	
Pension/profit sharing plan	
Social Security payroll taxes	
Unemployment payroll taxes	
Optometric services, eyewear, and prescription lenses provided for employees	
Paid holidays	
Paid vacations	
Sick leave	
Uniform allowance	
Continuing education costs (tuition, transportation, lodging, and meals)	
Professional dues and subscriptions	
Other	

Delete those benefits that are not applicable and add others, such as 401K plan benefits, if they are part of an employee's salary package.

Then, total up the *value* of each employee's salary and benefits. In most cases, it is substantially higher than the person's take-home pay.

REALITY CHECK

C. J. Cranny, author of *Job Satisfaction: How People Feel about Their Jobs and How It Affects Their Performance* (Lexington Books, 1992), says that employee satisfaction is "a function of the difference between what employees want or think they should get, and what they're really getting." The problem often is that many employees simply don't know what they're getting. The Total Pay Statement is meant to close that gap. It's also an excellent tool for employee recruitment and retention.

163 Equity theory

Equity theory states that when employees feel underpaid, they will find a way to rectify the situation. The most obvious: Quit or ask for a raise. Other ways potentially more detrimental to your practice include attempts to make one's job more rewarding in *non-financial ways*, such as socializing with co-workers, taking long breaks, and making personal phone calls. It may include slowing down at work and becoming less productive and attentive to details (telltale sign: three people are needed to do the job of two). If feelings run deeper, it may result in "white collar crime," such as stealing, just to "even the score."

What employees do, according to equity theory, is compare what is called their *job inputs* (education, skills, experience, responsibility, productivity, years on the job) and *job outputs* (salary and benefits) with *those of co-workers*. When this ratio is out of balance, a sense of *inequity* is experienced. It happens, for example, when an employee thinks his or her job is more difficult or demanding than that of a co-worker who is paid the same, let alone a *higher salary*.

"The lack of *written job descriptions* often results in some employees doing more (or less) than they were initially hired to do," says David Goodnight, D.V.M., M.B.A., and executive vice president of business development for Veterinary Pet Insurance. "For a variety of reasons," he adds, "it just happens, and in time, the overworked person is likely to sense an inequity. Periodic performance reviews (including two-way dialogue about the job, the employee's job performance, and the compensation) will uncover such a problem before it becomes full-blown. The solution: Adjust workloads, salaries, or benefits and, if necessary, hire additional people—even if it means increasing overhead. In the end, you'll have greatly improved employee morale, productivity, and practice growth."

164 Is a counteroffer the answer?

The dilemma: A key employee gives notice that she is leaving to take another job for more money. Do you make a counteroffer to persuade her to stay?

In speaking with a wide range of professionals and office managers, the consensus seems to be "No." The reason: The problems caused by counteroffers often outweigh the benefits. For example, if concessions are made and the employee stays, it may lead to resentment among other employees who feel they too deserve a raise, additional perks, a change in work schedule, or whatever. Worse yet, a counteroffer to a departing employee may lead to a chain reaction, prompting other employees to use the same tactic to gain concessions.

In addition, if the departing employee has repeatedly asked for a raise and been denied it, she may resent the lengths to which she had to go (i.e., giving notice) to finally get the raise she felt all along she deserved. At the same time, you may resent having to make such a concession under duress. Resentment on either side, let alone *on both sides,* is sure to erode employer-employee relations and the spirit of teamwork so necessary in a high-performance optometric practice.

REALITY CHECK

The one exception is a key employee who is critical to the day-to-day operation of the practice. In the long run, it may cost more to *replace* the person than to *retain* him or her. Consider making a counteroffer in such a case and take a chance that the aftermath will be smooth sailing.

165 Maintain alumni relations

Rather than lose touch with former staff members, Phillip E. Bly, D.D.S., Indianapolis, IN, started an alumni-relations program so employees who have shared work experiences over the years can stay in touch. He coordinates periodic get-togethers of current and former staff members. The group usually meets for a luncheon in a private dining room at a local country club or hotel. On other occasions, the employees and their spouses gather for a picnic, a swim, bowling, or a Christmas party.

The get-togethers, Dr. Bly says, are fun and provide some unexpected fringe benefits to his practice. For example, most of these former employees remain with the practice as patients, bringing, in some cases, their spouses and children. Many continue to be active referral sources for the practice. On occasion, when Dr. Bly is short-handed, the former employees fill in on an emergency basis and are glad to help out. In fact, some of them say that being back in the practice is like "old home week."

Although not all of your former employees will want or be able to attend such alumni activities, many will. Those who do will benefit from the ongoing relationships.

166 Conduct performance reviews

Studies show that a high percentage of professional and clerical employees are in the dark about how they're doing on the job or how they can do better simply because they've never been told and have no way of knowing.

One result is that exceptional employees are unaware of their strengths and may or may not be consistent in what they do or how they do it. Those who feel their efforts are unnoticed and unappreciated may become demotivated or, worse, start looking for another job.

Another result is that marginal employees are unaware of their shortcomings and may assume that silence means approval (i.e., "If the doctor didn't like the way I do things, he would tell me").

Either way, you lose.

One solution to this communication gap is the *performance review.* It has been defined as a two-way dialogue between employer and employee about the latter's past, present, and future job performance. It includes a discussion of such matters as

• Recognition of good work
• Clarification of job responsibilities and priorities
• Suggestions for improvement—on both sides
• Agreement on how and by when such improvements will be made

Such discussions let people know how their performance on the job compares with your expectations. This helps employees identify their strengths, develop their talents, and enjoy their work.

ACTION STEPS

Before You Discuss the Person, Discuss the Job Itself. You may have different ideas about the exact nature of each job than your employees do. If you have a written job description, review it together to see if it needs revision. Then, ask such questions as

Do we agree on what your job is?

Which do you think are the most important elements of your job? Do we agree on these?

Do we agree on the standards by which your work will be evaluated?

Ask Before You Tell. Instead of *telling* employees what you think of their work, *ask* them (individually) to tell you what they think they have done well and what they would like to do better. Many criticize themselves more readily than they accept criticism from you. In fact, they may judge themselves more harshly than you would. The following questions may help facilitate the discussion:

What do you think are your greatest strengths?

In which areas do you feel less competent?

Do you feel you are becoming more competent as time goes by? If so, in what ways?

Is there any way that someone could help you do a better job?
Do I do anything that makes your job harder?

Management expert Peter Drucker says, "The greatest boost to productivity would be for managers to ask, 'What do we do in this organization that helps you do the job you're being paid for—and what do we do that hampers you?'"

Keep Criticism Impersonal by Discussing "Job Performance" Only. For example, you can call a person "irresponsible," or you can say, "this job was to be completed by the 15th and it wasn't done until the 18th." The first statement is opinion and open to question. The second is fact.

Determine the Cause of Poor Performance. Encourage employees to analyze problems by asking, "That's an unusual number of billing errors. What happened?" or "How can we prevent this from happening in the future?" Then, wait for an answer.

Agree on a Plan of Action. The improvement you want in an employee's work habits or performance can occur only when you both perceive the problem in the same way and agree on the means and a timetable for solving it.

Start with your own recommendation—or better yet, invite your employees to tell you how they would like to develop themselves and what help, if any, they would like from you. Be specific. Set deadlines. Then, put this "action plan" on paper as a form of "contract" between you and your employee. Such commitment gets better results than vague promises. The action plan also serves as a benchmark against which future progress (or, if necessary, grounds for dismissal) can be measured.

REALITY CHECK

Don't be surprised if employees say, "This is the first time since the day I was hired that anyone has ever sat down and asked my view of things" and then *thank you* for taking the time to do it.

167 Upward communication

The fact that you never hear job-related complaints from employees doesn't necessarily mean everyone is happy. Many employees are reluctant to speak up when they dislike something about their work or the way they are treated by their boss. Some are timid or afraid. Others think speaking up would be a waste of time because nothing would change if they did. So, they talk among themselves, their families, and perhaps with patients as well, about the things that bother them about the practice, and the problems continue.

Eventually, this lack of communication takes its toll. Unhappy people do not perform as well as those who like their jobs. They are not as interested in what they do or how well they do it. They tend to be slower, perhaps more careless, and they are not as pleasant. In time, it begins to affect everyone's morale, patients included.

Firing unhappy employees is not the answer. Effective management and motivation of people depend on good communication— *upward* as well as downward.

Downward communication takes place when the doctor does the talking and the staff listens. Upward communication is the just the opposite: The staff talks, the *doctor* listens.

Upward communication is the only way optometrists can ascertain the level of employee morale and job satisfaction, and what changes, if any, are needed to improve it. It is also the key to discovering what impact their management style has on others.

Upward communication is only meaningful if employees are free to "tell it like it is" and are confident the doctor will listen with an open mind. If they are concerned that their job security or future raises might in any way be threatened by what they say, it's understandable (and predictable) that they'll say only what they think the doctor *wants* to hear, and the problems will continue.

One technique for initiating upward communication in an optometric practice is the Employee Survey. It's widely used as a management tool in industry to learn what employees think of their jobs, working conditions, quality of supervision, compensation, co-workers, opportunities for advancement, and other factors.

The advantage of the Employee Survey is that many employees are more comfortable expressing themselves *anonymously* on paper than they are in person. This greatly improves the chances of getting truthful results.

The following is a composite of Employee Surveys used in a wide variety of health care professions. Use or modify it for your particular situation. Add additional questions. And leave space for employees to elaborate on their answers.

Employee Survey	Strongly Agree	Agree	Disagree	Strongly Disagree
1) The people I work with help each other out when someone falls behind or gets in a tight spot.				
2) When changes are made that affect me, I am usually told the reasons for the changes.				
3) The doctor really tries to get our ideas about things.				
4) The doctor's review of my performance gives me a clear picture of how I'm doing on the job.				
5) The practice could benefit from more frequent staff meetings.				
6) My job is a satisfactory challenge to me.				
7) Our staff meetings are a waste of time.				
8) If I have a complaint, I feel free to tell the doctor about it.				
9) The doctor has always been fair in dealing with me.				
10) I look forward to coming to work.				
11) The doctor lets us know exactly what's expected of us.				
12) There's too much pressure in my job.				
13) Some of the working conditions here need to be changed.				
14) I'm paid fairly compared with other employees.				
15) My job has not turned out to be as it was described to me when I was hired.				

Employee Survey	Strongly Agree	Agree	Disagree	Strongly Disagree
16) I have all the authority I need to perform my job properly.				
17) I have been properly trained to do my job.				
18) I am very much underpaid for the work I do.				
19) I have the right equipment and materials to do my job well.				
20) The office policies are clearly spelled out.				
21) I am given the opportunity to learn and grow in my job.				
22) I feel my efforts to do a good job are appreciated.				
23) I enjoy working with the people here.				
24) The doctor lets me know in a fair and constructive manner when I have done something wrong.				
25) The hours of work are satisfactory.				
26) Our productivity sometimes suffers from lack of organization and planning.				
27) I think some good may come out of completing this survey.				

Optional: The reason I feel as I do about question No.____ is:_____

_____

What I think should be done about it is: _____

REALITY CHECK

Will such a survey open a can of worms? Create more problems than it solves? The answer is no. Problems either do or do not already exist. Ignoring them will not make them go away: It may, in fact, make them *worse*, lead to deep resentment, and cause a capable person to quit.

Evidence indicates that the attitude of employees tends to improve when they are given an opportunity to speak their minds. It's why such surveys are so widely used in industry.

168 Prevent staff burnout

Job burnout is a form of work-related stress that affects the disposition and productivity of everyone in the office. Burned-out employees grow more and more negative about their jobs, doing the bare minimum required to get the job done. Often they become irritable toward co-workers, employers, and even patients. They are late for work, call in sick more often, and may quit their jobs.

On the surface, burnout looks like an employee problem.

Christina Maslach, Ph.D., professor of psychology, University of California, Berkeley, says burnout is caused as much by the job and the way people are managed as it is by an employee's personality.[7]

The first step in preventing burnout is to understand what causes it. The following are three stress-producing scenarios commonly found in optometric practices:

WORK OVERLOAD

With the demands of increasing paperwork, patients to see, prescriptions to process, *and* the need for greater productivity, it's not uncommon to hear employees say, "There's just too much work to do and never enough time. I don't know where to start."

REALITY CHECK

A study by the Families and Work Institute asked 1,003 working adults who were not self-employed whether they felt overworked. Twenty-eight percent reported they feel overworked often or very often. Another 28% said they feel overwhelmed by the amount of work they have to complete. The percentages increased substantially when asked whether they *sometimes* experienced these feelings (54% and 55%, respectively).

How do these feelings have an impact on staff members? The study indicates that the more overworked employees feel, the more likely they are to make mistakes at work, feel angry toward their employers, resent co-workers who do not work as hard, and look for a new job, in addition to the toll these feelings take on their health and home life. What the study did not mention was that overworked employees who are angry and resentful are unlikely to be friendly and attentive to patients.[8]

ROLE CONFLICT

Mixed messages are the problem in this case. An example is an optometrist who stresses that employees should be friendly and helpful to patients, *while at the same time* expects them to handle an increased workload. That is a tough assignment. If a bottleneck occurs on a busy day, which "role" takes precedence?

ROLE AMBIGUITY

When employees are uncertain about exactly what is expected of them on a day-to-day basis, they experience stress. As previously mentioned, the complaint, "My job has not turned out to be the way it was described to me when I was hired" is a common one (No. 15 on the Employee Survey).

ACTION STEPS

How does one resolve these stressful, workplace situations? The first step: Identify the problem. The Performance Review and/or Employee Survey may be helpful.

Next, with input from employees, develop detailed written job descriptions that spell out as completely as possible what is expected of each employee. If job descriptions already exist, review and update them to reflect any changes that have occurred because of practice growth, managed care, increased delegation, new personnel, etc. Then, with one-on-one input from each person, prioritize each task.

Consider trade-offs of job responsibilities between employees to even out everyone's workload, perhaps enabling each person to do more of what he or she likes doing.

Another option: Hire part-time employees to alleviate the workload of overburdened employees (discussed in Chapter 9).

169 Dilemma of the inflexible, long-term employee

A surprising number of successful practices are impacted by a single employee who is out of step with everyone else but, for various reasons, remains on the payroll. Recent complaints I've heard include the following:

- "Our receptionist (of 11 years) refuses to change her outdated ways of doing things. The practice has grown, but she hasn't."
- "My clinical technician (of 7 years) has become so overbearing and rude to patients and other staff members that it has created unbearable stress in the office."
- "Our optician (of 5 years) thinks he knows everything. If I say anything about his work, he rolls his eyes and there's often a scene."

What typically complicates these situations is that these employees are *not* thought to be totally unsatisfactory. Frequently, they're passable, if not good, at some aspects of their jobs and less than satisfactory in other aspects.

The reasons given by optometrists for not firing such employees are often similar: a sense of obligation ("because of his or her many years of service") or kindness ("she needs the job"), or because "I dread having to fire him."

If you're faced with such a dilemma, the question to consider is "To whom do you owe what?" What do you owe a long-term employee who will not change? What do you owe your patients, associates, and other staff members who have to contend with such behavior? And what do you owe *yourself* in this situation? How troubling is it for you?

If you have conducted periodic performance reviews with such employees, given fair warnings to those who need to change, documented such discussions, and have seen no improvement, it may be time to let them go.

170 Management's most unpleasant task

The most unpleasant and disliked task of practice management is having to fire an employee. Most optometrists detest the job.

The first thing to remember is that there's no way to make a dismissal pleasant. You can only minimize the pain and hostility.

HARD-LEARNED LESSONS ABOUT FIRING EMPLOYEES

- Always fire someone face to face. The job can't be delegated any more than it can be postponed.
- Once you make the decision, "get 'em out quick." That's the overwhelming recommendation of the many personnel specialists I've asked about the timing of an employee's dismissal. The end of the day is preferred to avoid embarrassment for the employee. Mondays are preferred to Fridays so the person can go out on a Tuesday to look for other work, rather than stew about it on the weekend.
- Should you tell the employee the reasons for your decision or gloss over them? Most personnel managers advocate an explanation somewhere between the two extremes. They advise giving the employee enough information to show your decision was not arbitrary, but not so much detail as to destroy the person's self-esteem in the process.
- Stick to facts rather than feelings. Your opinions about a person's "attitude" or "personality" are debatable and accomplish little except to inflict pain.
- To avoid lawsuits claiming a wrongful dismissal, document everything as it occurs. When a problem is severe enough to require a warning, put it in writing, date it, and have the employee sign it. If it becomes necessary, this paper trail will provide a sound basis for a subsequent firing decision.
- Adopt a low-key approach that the employee is just not right for your practice, in that job, at this time. Do not dwell on shortcomings: Simply express disappointment that things have not changed since the last performance review, and that you have no alternative but to terminate employment. Acknowledge the person's capabili-

ties and strong points. If appropriate, express regret that you don't have a job opening more suited to the person's qualifications, and let it go at that.

171 Exit interviews

Ever wonder about the level of morale among your employees, or how they view their jobs, co-workers, and the day-to-day management of your practice? The answers could be helpful in improving productivity and practice growth.

Interviews with departing employees, called *exit interviews*, can often yield information that, for a variety of reasons, employees are reluctant to tell you while still on the job.

TESTED TIP

To get honest feedback, assure departing employees of complete confidentiality and that what they say during the exit interview will not, in any way, be held against them (e.g., if they ask for a reference).

SUGGESTED QUESTIONS

- Are there any specific features of your new job that you feel were lacking in your job here?
- What did you think about the features of your job here, such as salary, benefits, supervision, and office policies?
- What did you like best about your job here? What did you dislike about it?
- What suggestions do you have for us to make our office a better place to work?
- Were you satisfied or dissatisfied with the office environment? Are changes needed in the working space, lighting, heating, or air conditioning?
- How about the working conditions? Did you feel overworked? Underused? Were you under unusual stress?
- What were your real reasons for leaving our office? (Consider probing for the *critical factor* with follow-up questions such as "What

was the straw that broke the camel's back? When did you decide you wanted a different job?")

• Would you recommend our office as a good place to work?

All of these questions may not fit each departing employee, so pick and choose as the situation warrants. During the questioning, it's best to be empathetic and nonjudgmental. Comments such as "I wasn't aware of that; please go on" or "That's an interesting point; could you give me more details?" encourage the employee to speak openly.

REALITY CHECK

It's important to remember that departing employees are also "ambassadors" for your practice, whether you wish them to be or not. Even if they encountered several months of rough going before leaving, if the parting was amicable, they will be more inclined to speak favorably about the practice.

FROM THE SUCCESS FILES

"The more I tried to educate my staff about promptness and perfection," admits ophthalmologist, Dahlia Hirsch, M.D., Bel Air, MD, "the worse the situation became. It wasn't because of the message, but how I delivered it. I often didn't appreciate what my employees did. I only noticed what they didn't or couldn't do. I was impatient. Sometimes I corrected them right in front of patients. My wake-up call came one day when all four of my employees quit. We went to lunch, which became an exit interview of sorts, and I asked them why they were quitting. I learned (painfully) that I was the reason. That lunch," she adds, "was the most valuable consultation I ever had. I realized that if I didn't change some patterns, I would have constant turnover."[9]

---

172   Hard-learned lessons about personnel management

• James Autry said, "Good management is largely a matter of love. Or if you're uncomfortable with that word, call it caring, because proper management involves caring for people, not manipulating them."

- Coddle your employees. Without them, you may not have a practice. If necessary, pay them before you pay yourself. Give them benefits you would not take for yourself. Spoil them and empower them in every way possible.
- People's on-the-job performance and productivity tend to improve when they know what is expected of them and receive periodic feedback about their work.
- "It's not the people you fire who make your life miserable, it's those you don't"(Harvey Mackay, *Swim with the Sharks*, William Morrow & Co. Inc., 1988).
- The way you treat your employees is the way they will treat your patients.

Notes

1. How to Close the Revolving Door of Employee Turnover. *Blair/McGill Advisory*, June 2001, 4.
2. Hayes J. Beyond School. *Optometric Management*, August 2001, 32,34.
3. West WD. Delegation and Patient Education. *Contact Lens Spectrum*, April 2001, 50.
4. Borish IM. Delegation = Survival. *Optometric Economics*, September 1992, 30–31.
5. Gailmard NB. Write Stuff. *Optometric Management*, November 2001, 75–78.
6. Porter MA. Rehabilitating the Older Injured Worker. *Work*, Fall 1991, 54–60.
7. Maslach C, Leiter M. *The Truth about Burnout: How Organizations Cause Stress and What to Do about It.* San Francisco: Jossey-Bass, 1997.
8. Galinsky E, Kim SS, Bond JT. Feeling Overworked: When Work Becomes Too Much. *Families and Work Institute*, 2001, 6,11.
9. Hirsch D. Practice Management: How to Rediscover the Person in the Patient. *Review of Optometry*, July 1999.

11

How to Keep Staff Motivation in High Gear

What is it that makes staff members go out of their way to be friendly to patients? Attend continuing education courses to improve their knowledge and skills? Pitch in and help a co-worker who is behind in his or her work? Recommend their friends to your practice? These are *discretionary acts* performed by high-performance employees who feel a strong obligation to do what's "right" for patients, co-workers, and the practice itself.

173 Compliance, cooperation, and commitment

For purposes of discussion, let us divide employees into three basic groups:

- *Compliant* employees do only what they have to do to get by, avoid criticism, and keep their jobs. Many think of their work as "just a job."
- *Cooperative* employees go a step further. They are more highly motivated to do what you want and are more agreeable about it.
- *Committed* employees have an intense, *inner desire* to do the very best job possible. They are self-starters, not limited by a job description, and often do more than is expected of them, more than they are paid to do. In a word, they *like* coming to work. It is more than "just a job."

"A committed employee," says consultant David L. Stum, Ph.D., "is one who is a team player, who is willing to make personal sacrifices for the good of the company, who believes in the company's product, who will recommend the company as among the best places to work, and who is prepared to stay at the company for at least the next several years, even if offered a modest increase elsewhere."[1]

174 Ask for commitment, not loyalty

"At Brush-Wellman Inc., we are asking for the commitment—not loyalty of employees," says Daniel Skoch, vice president of human resources. "Commitment requires an agreement to do something; loyalty implies being blindly faithful to a duty or obligation. Thus, we have begun to tell our employees:

'We will help you grow and develop. We will provide you opportunities to learn, to be involved, to practice new skills, to have responsibility, to be respected and valued, and to be rewarded and recognized for your contributions. In return, we seek your commitment to our company's mission. We cannot guarantee what is going to happen in the future, but if it doesn't work out, you will leave here a more talented, responsible, self-confident, and employable person.'

"As a result," says Mr. Skoch, "we believe that our employees recognize that their personal needs for security, growth opportunities, and job satisfaction can link up very well with the company's need for employees who are willing to continually learn, and be adaptable and self-supervising. This linking will provide us with a competitive advantage and our employees with their best opportunity for personal security."[2]

What accounts for such commitment? Much of it is innate. If you spot it in a job candidate, hire the person. Commitment can also be nurtured by a management style that's responsive to employees' job-related needs—so let's start with those.

175 Motivation Inventory

Place an X next to the *five job-related needs* in the following list that you believe are most important in motivating the *one employee* in your office you would most like to motivate:

1. Assurance of regular employment
2. Satisfactory working conditions
3. Suitable rest periods and coffee breaks
4. Adequate vacation arrangements and holidays
5. Good pay
6. Having the goals and objectives of the practice spelled out so I know where we are headed
7. A written job description so I know what is expected of me
8. Periodic performance reviews so I know how I am doing
9. Health insurance and other fringe benefits
10. The avoidance of criticism for doing an inadequate job
11. Maintenance of adequate living standards for my family
12. Being told by the doctor that I'm doing a good job
13. Getting along with co-workers
14. Participation in management activities
15. Involvement in decisions affecting my work
16. Feeling that my job is important
17. Respect for me as a person and/or a professional at my job
18. Have more autonomy on the job
19. Have more job responsibilities
20. Interesting work
21. Opportunities to do work that is challenging
22. Chance for self-development and improvement
23. Others

REALITY CHECK

Seminar audiences typically struggle with this Motivation Inventory simply because it is difficult for them to know their employees' job-related needs unless they have discussed the subject with them.

ACTION STEP

What we need to do is identify employees' job-related needs and then make their jobs so satisfying that they will want, *really want*, to do their best, or as Bob Townsend, former CEO of Avis said, "Create the kind of environment that pays people to bring their brains to work."

176 Learn employees' job-related needs

There are several ways to learn about such needs:

- Ideally, the initial job interview uncovers an applicant's job-related needs. The underlying purpose of many of the interview questions listed in Chapter 9 is to help you ascertain if you have the right person for the right job in your office (e.g., "What about your last job did you like most? Least?").

REALITY CHECK

Jack Welch, former chairman and CEO of General Electric, claims that 90% of good management is about getting the right people in the right jobs.[3]

- Consider asking current employees similar questions to identify their job-related needs. In this case, put them in writing. Give them time to think about their answers; perhaps discuss them with someone else. Explain also that if they'd like to do so, you'll schedule a one-on-one conference to discuss the results. Such questions might include the following:
  - What part of your job do you like best—and why?
  - Are there additional things you would like to be doing?
  - What, if anything, frustrates you about your job?
  - What is there about your job (if anything) that you would like changed to help you get more of what you want from your work?

- The Motivation Inventory, although not intended for this purpose, can be used.

- Performance Reviews (see Chapter 10) are a more formal, in-depth way to learn employees' job-related needs.

Having identified job-related needs, the next step is to help employees get more of what they want from their work.

It's not possible to discuss all of these job-related needs in a single chapter. A few, such as job descriptions and performance reviews (No. 7 and No. 8 in the Motivation Inventory, respectively), were discussed in the last chapter. Let us consider a few others in the following sections.

177 Satisfactory working conditions (No. 2, Motivation Inventory)

Louis Harris did a survey of office workers regarding their "work environment." Not surprisingly, the factor considered most important was "good lighting." Number two was "comfortable seating"—again, not surprising considering that back ailments affect 60–80% of the population and are the number two cause of absenteeism. (Number one is the common cold.)

What *is* surprising is how often employees complain about an "uncomfortable chair in which I have to sit all day!"

REALITY CHECK

Uncomfortable chairs contribute to more frequent stretch breaks, employee errors, and lower job satisfaction—*especially if employees complain about the problem and nothing is done.*

Another related source of complaints: office equipment and ophthalmic instruments that are out of date, frequently require repair, and that need to be replaced.

The inference in both cases: "You and your work are not important enough to remedy the situation."

REALITY CHECK

How friendly, understanding, or helpful are such demotivated employees going to be when dealing with patients? As the old saying goes: What goes around, comes around.

ACTION STEPS

Replace that which needs to be replaced and *empower* the employee who uses the chair or equipment on a daily basis to recommend (or buy outright) what's needed.

There are of course, degrees of empowerment. Decide which is most appropriate, based on the nature of the task and the abilities of the employee. For example, you can tell an employee any one of the following:

- Investigate the situation. Report back to me. I'll decide.
- Investigate. Make recommendations. I'll decide.
- Investigate. Decide. Let me have final approval.
- Take action. Let me know what you did.
- Whatever you do is OK with me.

REALITY CHECK

Empowerment to make such recommendations or decisions is very satisfying to people with the job-related need for "involvement in decisions affecting my work" (No. 15 in the Motivation Inventory) and who seek more on-the-job responsibility and authority. In fact, many would consider it insulting *not* to be consulted in such matters.

A complaint I often hear from disgruntled employees: "I'm treated as if I don't have a brain in my head."

178 Need for interesting work (No. 20, Motivation Inventory)

When asked, "What makes a job satisfying?" 30,000 readers of *Working Woman* magazine ranked "interesting and challenging work" number one.[4]

REALITY CHECK

It has been said that 75% of jobs can be learned in 3 years. For some people, doing the same thing every day is fine. For others, it results in boredom.

One of the best ways to make work more interesting is to give people with this need a chance to grow on the job. Tackle tasks that require what industrial psychologists call *s-t-r-e-t-c-h*. The principle involved: *The competence of most people is increased when given a challenge.* It's the same principle as playing a sport with someone who's a *little* better at it than you. It could be ping-pong, dancing, or Scrabble—it's motivational. Makes you perform better. That's s-t-r-e-t-c-h. And, because you play better, you also have a *sense of achievement.*

HARD-LEARNED LESSONS

It's achievement that leads to motivation—not the other way around. You see it in the "high-fives" that athletes trade after scoring a touchdown or hitting a home run. You see it in the expression of someone on a diet who discovers, after weeks of self-discipline, that he has lost 5 pounds.

The point is that if you want to motivate employees, don't lecture them. Don't threaten them with dismissal if they fail to improve. Instead, provide *s-t-r-e-t-c-h* and opportunities for achievement.

ACTION STEPS

Ask employees what specific knowledge and skills they'd like to learn. Then, design a program that incorporates the needs of individuals as well as the practice itself.

179 Additional opportunities for growth

For employees interested in personal and professional growth, consider the following:

- *Job rotation*: Gives employees an opportunity to try different jobs in the office. Provides a change of pace. Helps everyone better understand the demands of each other's jobs. Promotes teamwork. And, in the event of an "emergency," enables a cross-trained person to "fill in," if only on a limited basis.
- *On the-job training*: Enables employees to upgrade their job skills by working with someone more experienced or knowledgeable.
- *Continuing education programs*: Enables employees to learn new clinical, optical, and office-related skills.

- *Job enrichment*: Involves additional responsibilities such as buying frames for the dispensary, purchasing equipment, leading staff meetings, interviewing job applicants, and doing marketing research.
- *Participative management*: Includes participation in S.W.O.T. analysis, long-range strategic planning for the practice.

FROM THE SUCCESS FILES

Nancy G. Torgerson, O.D., F.C.O.V.D., Lynnwood, WA, schedules in-office training for her 7 vision therapists once a week, for an hour and a half (9:30–11:00 a.m.). Among the topics: amblyopia, strabismus, visual thinking, visual memory, directionality, laterality, and spatial relationships.

Each therapist-in-training becomes an associate of the Optometric Extension Program Foundation (http://www.oep.org) and an Optometric Vision Therapist Technician in the College of Optometrists in Vision Development (http://www.covd.org) and begins the process of becoming certified. These organizations give them access to journals, books, newsletters, and education. Attending Optometric Extension Program Foundation regional clinical seminars, congresses, and the College of Optometrists in Vision Development Annual Meeting provides additional opportunities to grow and network, enjoy camaraderie, and remain excited about their field.

"This training pays off in many ways," says Dr. Torgerson. "The staff is more knowledgeable; able to do more for patients *and* provide better care. This in turn delights patients and parents. Makes them excited about our office.

"Hearing patients rave about the practice is great for our team spirit," she adds. "Staff morale is great."

180 Hard-learned lessons about staff training

- An article in *Fortune* entitled "Managing for the Slowdown" stresses the importance of quality employees: "We hope it's no longer necessary to argue that this is increasingly your company's only source of competitive advantage. . . . Getting the best people and making them better is in the DNA of the most successful companies."[5]

- Staff training is most appealing to people who have such job-related needs as more job responsibilities, interesting work, opportunities to do work that is challenging, and chance for self-development and improvement (Nos. 19–22 in the Motivation Inventory).

- Training someone who wishes only a paycheck is as pointless and self-defeating as placing someone with a desire for professional growth in a repetitive, dead-end job.

- Surprisingly, some optometrists say they cannot afford to train because of the expense and because better-trained, more highly skilled employees may decide to leave for better opportunities. That's true, but training new employees and having them leave is not nearly as bad as *not* training them and having them stay.

181 Need for appreciation (No. 12, Motivation Inventory)

Psychologist William James wrote, "The deepest principle in human nature is the craving to be appreciated." Notice that he didn't say "wish" or "desire," or even "longing." He said *craving*.

Finding something nice to say about others may seem trivial, but it satisfies a universal hunger. Unfortunately, people who feel appreciation often fail to express it. They become inhibited, forgetful, and busy with other day-to-day priorities.

Many optometric employees I've interviewed feel most thwarted and frustrated about their work because of a lack of appreciation. Included are those who do above-average work but receive no special recognition or appreciation. Many have said, "The only time I get any feedback about my work is when I make a mistake." They also believe that their efforts to do a good job are never even *noticed*, let alone appreciated.

Some doctors mistakenly assume their employees' need for appreciation can be *internally* met ("She knows she does a good job"). Even if that were true, a verbal pat on the back or a written note of thanks for a "job well done" provides the kind of psychological satisfaction for which there is absolutely no substitute.

When President Reagan wrote "Very Good" on the draft of a speech prepared by speechwriter Peggy Noonan, she cut the words out, taped them to her blouse, and wore them all day.

The list of candidates for appreciation is endless if you stop and think of the many people who contribute to the success of your practice. For a start, thank your staff for doing such a great job—I guarantee it will make their day. By expressing appreciation, you may start a chain reaction. Praise begets praise. People will like you more for saying kind things, and you will feel good for having said them.

182 The feedback gap

In the course of conducting seminars for a wide range of professional groups, I've asked more than 1,000 doctors to consider the following statement: *I let my employees know when they're doing a good job*, and then rate themselves on a scale of 1 to 5 (1 = never; 5 = always). The average response: 4.4.

So far, so good.

At these same seminars, I've also asked *staff members* to consider the statement: *The doctor lets me know when I'm doing a good job*, using the same rating scale. The average response: only 1.7.

The difference between the amount of positive feedback doctors *say* they give their employees and the amount employees say they *get* is what I call the *feedback gap*. Often, it is the underlying cause of employee resentment, diminished productivity, and turnover.

TESTED TIP

One clue to a job applicant's need for appreciation is his or her answer to the question, "In your last job, did you receive the recognition and appreciation you felt you deserved?"

183 How to multiply the power of your appreciation

According to management consultant and author Rosabeth Moss Kanter, "Saying thank you in public and perhaps giving a tangible gift along with it, has multiple functions beyond simple courtesy. To the employee, it signifies someone has noticed and cares. What is the point," she says, "of going all out to do something special if no one notices and it does not seem to make one whit of difference? To the rest of the organization, recognition creates role models—*heroes*—and communicates the standard: These are the kinds of things that constitute good performance around here."[6]

FROM THE SUCCESS FILES

Jim Bacon, D.V.M., Somerset, NJ, has exceptionally enthusiastic and loyal employees. One of the reasons is his sincere effort to let his staff know how much they are appreciated. "We send roses to each staff member on Valentine's Day," he explains. "We show gratitude for what they do throughout the year with a large fruit basket and bottle of wine at Thanksgiving. This past year for Secretaries' Day, we surprised everyone with $50 gift certificates, good at any of the stores in one of the area's largest shopping malls. We have yearly picnics, going-away dinners for departing staff members, and a year-end dinner with spouses at a fine restaurant. We use the Christmas party as an opportunity to present staff members who have reached 10 years of service during the previous year with a special gift, usually a weekend for two at one of the nearby resorts."

ACTION STEPS

A simple sentence will get you started: "That was a first-class job you did" or "I hear such nice things from patients about you" or "I'm glad you're on the team."

Go ahead. Make someone's day!

184 Hard-learned lessons about appreciation

- *Appreciation* results in short-term motivation.
- *Achievement* leads to long-term motivation.

People differ in what they want to be applauded and appreciated for, says Marc Talbin, CEO of a high-tech staffing consulting company in Sunnyvale, CA, depending on what personal qualities and talents they're most proud of. "My experience in managing people is they're all different," he says. "Some want to be recognized for the quality of their work, some for the quantity of their work. Some people want to be recognized for their cheerful attitude and their ability to spread their cheerful attitude. Some like to be recognized individually; others want to be recognized in groups. No one has ever said, 'Just recognize me for anything I do well.'" To identify which parts of individual employees' egos need scratching, Albin takes an unconventional approach: He asks them.[7]

FROM THE SUCCESS FILES

An optometric assistant with whom I was speaking at a recent seminar was discussing a job offer she received from another practice. It offered her more money, but she turned it down. I asked her why.

"I can't leave this office," she said. "The doctor is a stickler for detail and demanding—but he's also considerate in many ways I'll never forget. When my husband and I recently vacationed in Bermuda, for example, we found on our arrival a tremendous bouquet of flowers in our room from him and his wife. He had remembered that this was where we had honeymooned."

Countless reports like this reinforce my conviction in the value of recognition and appreciation, not as a substitute for salary and fringe benefits, but as important supplements to them.

185 Group pride

You sense it the moment you walk in the front door of a high-performance optometric practice: The staff welcomes you to "our office." They speak of "our practice" and "our patients" with such obvious pride, joy, and enthusiasm that you know they have their hearts in their work, that what they do is more than "just a job."

How does it happen?

Dr. Rensis Likert of the University of Michigan's Research Center has found that high-performance organizations are invariably characterized by feelings of *group pride*. His studies indicate that a decisive factor in such cases is the degree to which people

- Meet and interact with one another
- Identify with one another
- Seek to achieve organizational goals through collaborative efforts

Championship teams do each of those things. The scientists, astronauts, and ground crews at NASA do them, as do the people in high-performance practices.

It starts at the top—with you—and even the simplest gesture can make a difference. For example, introducing a paraoptometric who is assisting you in the exam room to the patient—perhaps adding, "Linda's the best. We're lucky to have her"—sends a very different message than failing to acknowledge her.

How do you develop these feelings of group pride? One way is with staff meetings.

186 Lively, interactive staff meetings

If your staff meetings have become a waste of time, in which the participants sit in stony silence with their arms folded, contributing little if anything to the discussion and waiting for the meeting to end, give the following tips a try. They may revive the meetings by making them livelier, more interactive, more productive, and more fun.

- Ask your staff what they consider the best time for a meeting and pay them if it's not during regular office hours. (Asking staff members to stay late or come in early is not conducive to getting their best thinking.) If lunchtime is selected, make it your treat. You'll see the difference this one change will make in people's attitudes.
- Give advance notice of the date and the agenda of staff meetings, rather than catch people off-guard and unprepared. Encourage staff members to add appropriate topics of their own.
- Rotate the leadership of the meeting among everyone in the practice, on a volunteer basis. Make it a leadership *opportunity*, not an *obligation*.
- Stick to the agenda. If a real give-and-take discussion is the goal, the meeting leader should make short statements, not speeches. Pass

over minor points. Encourage participation. Avoid negativity. At the staff meetings held by Jan Wolf, D.V.M., Kenosha, WI, participants used "clickers" to signal someone who was being unnecessarily negative, long-winded, or otherwise out of order. It kept the discussion positive and on target.

- It's worth repeating: Do not allow staff meetings to become *gripe sessions*.
- Whenever possible, implement changes in office policies and procedures by *consensus*. People tend to be more supportive of decisions in which they have some input. They're also more interested in seeing a successful outcome than they are of decisions made by others and passed along to them to implement.
- Set a time limit and stick to it. If necessary, schedule another staff meeting. It's better to quit on a high note than to have people looking at their watches, waiting for the meeting to end.
- If you're the leader, spend more time *listening*—than talking.
- Close staff meetings with an idea from the office of Jim Lanier, O.D., Jacksonville, FL: "Each staff member compliments another who has helped make her job easier during the past month. This includes the doctors, office manager, and all staff positions."[8]
- Schedule staff meetings as often as they're needed and continue to be productive.

FROM THE SUCCESS FILES

- "In our practice," says Larry K. Wan, O.D., who practices in a multidoctor setting in Campbell, CA, "we have weekly meetings where we talk about new products, procedures, insurance forms, and the like."[9]
- "About once a month, we schedule luncheon programs that are conducted by reps from labs, distributors, or manufacturers," says Gary A. Osias, O.D., San Lorenzo, CA. "These reps are worth their weight in gold. They help our staff to more effectively present their products and answer patients' questions."

187   More secrets of successful staff meetings

- Periodically, hold staff meetings at which everyone *stands*. You'll be amazed how much can be accomplished in so little time.

- Have everyone bring to a meeting at least one idea to improve office décor, appointment scheduling, collections, or recalls.
- Have everyone bring to a meeting at least one idea to save time or money or needed office space.
- Award prizes for the best such ideas.
- Make it a practice, at least initially, to call on people who appear interested and attentive to help get the discussion under way, rather than those who avoid eye contact and indicate little interest in participating.
- Invite outside speakers, such as ophthalmologists, management consultants, sales representatives, laboratory personnel, and perhaps patients themselves to address the group.
- For a change of pace, show a videotape for in-service training or inspiration.
- Focus on a positive approach. There is a world of difference between "How can we work better as a team?" and "Why is there so much friction and back-stabbing in our office?"
- Beware of "idea killers" such as "We tried that once before and it didn't work" or "Our patients will never go for that."
- Always conclude meetings with one or more *decisions*. Don't leave everyone wondering: What did we decide? Where do we go next? Make sure a plan of action is spelled out with a schedule of implementation.
- Hold some meetings without the doctor(s): They often inhibit the proceedings.
- Hold some meetings away from the office.

188   Early-morning "huddles"

An *early-morning huddle* refers to mini-staff meetings, typically 5–10 minutes in length, held at the start of the business day. Among its purposes are the following:

- To review the highlights of the previous day, including what went particularly well and any compliments heard about staff members, the doctor(s), the service, or the practice in general. This discussion starts the day on a positive, upbeat note.

- To verify that prescriptions promised for the day are in-house and ready to be delivered.
- To organize the day's activities and anticipate, if possible, the special needs of the patients being seen that day. For example, "Mrs. Gumby is coming in at 11. Let's really try to make her smile." Or "Do any of today's patients have payments that are long overdue? If so, who will deal with the matter?"
- To learn if anyone needs help with anything on the day's schedule. Doing so acknowledges that a busy day is coming up. Proactively deals with problems. Creates an atmosphere of cooperation.

Among the benefits of early-morning huddles are the following:

- Eliminates "surprises" (the avoidable ones, anyway)
- Greatly improves office efficiency and patient relations
- Fosters teamwork

Optometrists and staff members who have early-morning huddles are invariably enthusiastic about them. Once the habit is developed, the day seems strangely empty without one.

189 Promote a culture of change

As you've undoubtedly surmised, creating a high-performance practice is not a set formula—it's a "mindset." That mindset must lead to constant innovation and change. It may be awkward at first, but eventually becomes a way of life in your practice.

Ask yourself: Do you embrace change? Do your staff members know you desire ongoing improvements? Is this something you think about and communicate to them?

FROM THE SUCCESS FILES

If change is overdue in your practice, consider holding what Gene M. Kangley, D.D.S., and his staff in Pompano Beach, FL, call a "How We Can Do It Better" meeting.

First, Dr. Kangley asks everyone in the office to submit a list of practice-related matters that need change and/or improvement. Two weeks before the meeting, a compiled list is circulated. I saw one with 13 items. Among them: security measures needed in the office and general building area, remodeling of the bathroom, medical emergency procedures, protocol for a new patient emergency visit, out-of-office public relations, and appointment scheduling.

The meetings are held quarterly on a Friday from 12:00 p.m. to 2:00 p.m. with a catered lunch. Follow-up meetings are held each Monday from 8:30 a.m. to 9:00 a.m. to monitor the progress of the agreed-upon changes and to review the week's schedule. It is a team approach to make change an *ongoing* process.

Last year, 577 employees of Bic Corporation's Milford, CT, factory, participating in workplace-improvement meetings, came up with 2,999 recommendations. Of these, 2,368 were implemented. This is no management gimmick to stroke workers' egos, says administrator Charles Tichy. Bic takes this program very seriously, viewing it as a way to spur morale and productivity and, ultimately, bolster corporate profits.[10]

Added Benefits.   Staff meetings not only boost productivity and profits; they also satisfy several of the important job-related needs in the Motivation Inventory: participation in management activities, involvement in decisions affecting my work, feeling my job is important, and respect for me as a person and/or a professional at my job (Nos. 14–17, respectively, in the Motivation Inventory).

In Summary.   To the extent you can identify and address the job-related needs of your employees, the more prone they will be to engage in what psychologists call *motivated behavior.*

190 Hard-learned lessons about motivating others

The question isn't "How do I get my employees do what I want them to do?" Rather, it's "How do I get my employees *to want to do* what I want them to do?"

- Trying to motivate others without understanding their job-related motivational needs is like trying to start a stalled car by kicking it.
- Football coaching great Lou Holtz said, "You can't pay people to excel. You can only pay them to show up."
- "Only satisfied customers can give people job security," writes Jack Welch, legendary CEO of General Electric. "Not companies."[11]
- Catch people in the act of doing something right—and tell them.
- Prove the significance of your employees. Make sure everyone on your staff feels famous for something. You want them to always have a reason to come to work.
- "People who work in a fulfilling work environment," says Tom Chappell, co-founder and president of personal-care product manufacturer Tom's of Maine, "where they feel both valued and respected, are more productive and loyal."[12]
- Almost without exception, good work that goes unnoticed and unappreciated tends to deteriorate.
- Some people would rather have *praise* than a *raise*.
- Money motivates people—but only up to a point.

REALITY CHECK

If you gave every employee a $1,000 raise starting tomorrow, how much harder would they work—and for how long?

Notes

1. Cole CL. Building Loyalty. *Workforce*, August 2000, 42–48.
2. Skoch DA. Ask for Commitment, Not Loyalty. *Industry Week*, November 21, 1994, 38.
3. Nelson B. Self-Motivation, Fact or Fiction. *Corporate Meetings & Incentives*, December 2001, 45.
4. Ciabattari J. The Biggest Mistake Top Managers Make. *Working Woman*, October 1996, 47–55.
5. Charan R, Colvin G. Managing for the Slowdown. *Fortune*, February 5, 2001, 78–88.
6. Nelson B. Celebrating Employee Achievements. *Potentials in Marketing*, June 1995, 10.
7. Buchanan L. Managing One-to-One. *Inc. Magazine*, October 2001, 83–89.

8. Christensen B. Staff Training + Delegation + Teamwork = Success. *Optometric Management*, March 2000, 104–105.
9. Satisfaction Guaranteed. Supplement to *Optometric Management*, September 2000, 3S–5S.
10. Flaherty J. Suggestions Rise from the Floors of U.S. Factories. *New York Times*, April 21, 2001, C1–C7.
11. Welch J. *Straight from the Gut.* New York: Warner Business Books, 2001.
12. Finnigan A. Benefits under Fire. *Working Woman*, July/August 2001, 54,56,58,78.

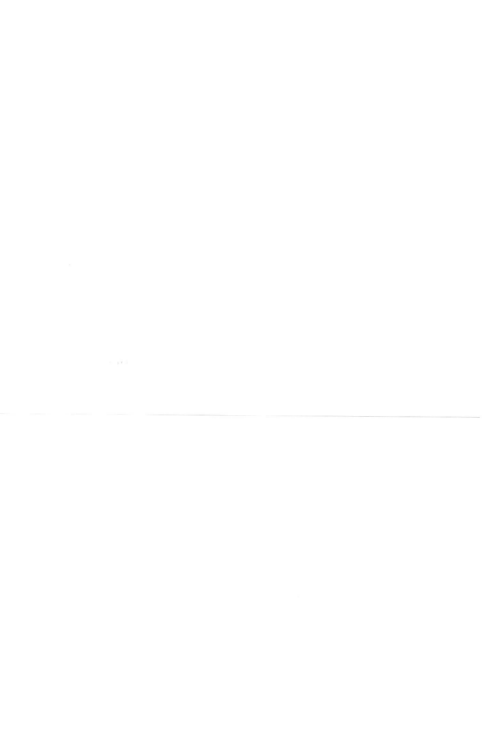

12

Secrets of Stress Management

How satisfying is your current practice? Does it often stress you out? Compromise your ideals? Give you the "blahs"?

I've met a surprising number of optometrists who, as the phrase goes, are looking good, but feeling bad. Something is missing: Their practices aren't as rewarding as they once were. Not as satisfying as they had hoped at this stage of their lives.

Fortunately, if you're not happy with your professional life, you have options—more today than ever. You can change your environment, your hours, your specialty, or even your location (from across town to across country). You can limit your practice to those aspects of practice you find most satisfying or add new ones. Join managed-care plans or reduce your dependency on them. Quit a salaried job and go off on your own. Join a multi-provider practice. Do part-time teaching or consulting. The possibilities are practically endless.

191 Clarify your basic values

Where do you start if you're unhappy with your practice? Career counselors advise that the first step is to clarify your basic values, those qualities you consider most worthwhile and important. Often, this type of evaluation results in the discovery that your values are not really yours at all; they've been imposed by others, telling you what you "should" do or the kind of practice you "should" have. Sometimes you just get caught up in what's happening at the moment, and may lose sight of the big picture.

GOLDEN HANDCUFF SYNDROME

A Texas O.D. told me about the mounting pressure he was getting from the optical chain at which he was employed to work faster, see more patients, and be more productive.

"It was getting to the point where I dreaded going to work," he said. "Yet, it was difficult to leave because it meant going out on my own, starting over, and initially at least, getting by on a greatly reduced income."

I call this double bind the *golden handcuff syndrome.*

After rank ordering his priorities, this optometrist decided to take the risk and make a fresh start in a more professional, personally satisfying type of practice. He's not (yet) making the income he previously was, but he's happier than he's been in years.

Being in a practice that is in conflict with your priorities—one that is all wrong for you—will, in time, lead to professional burnout. It's just a question of how long.

HARD-LEARNED LESSON

Something's wrong with the picture when you wake up on a Monday morning and wish it were Friday. It may be time to move on.

---

192 Instant vacations

Phaedrus, in the first century AD, said, "you will break the bow if you keep it always stretched."

He might well have been referring to the importance of what I call *instant vacations.* These are spur-of-the-moment "breaks" during hectic, nonstop periods of the day. Numerous studies have confirmed the rested body can do more than a tired one—and do it better.

FROM THE SUCCESS FILES

Ben Hara, D.P.M., a busy surgeon in Covina, CA, has for many years taken instant vacations in the form of mid-day naps, after a simple lunch ("the simpler, the better," he says). During this time, there are no phone calls and no visitors—no interruptions of any kind. "My mid-day nap," says Dr. Hara, "re-energizes me. Increases my productivity. Enables me to make two days out of one."

Instead of a mid-day nap, consider the following relaxation technique: sit or lie down in a comfortable place. Close your eyes. Become aware of your breathing. Breathe in through the nose to a count of four. Exhale through the mouth to a count of four. Picture in your mind a mountain meadow. Hear the rushing water. Picture the wildflowers. Feel the breeze against your face. Hear the sounds of birds, bees, and wind. With every intruding thought, repeat the phrase: "I am thinking of a mountain meadow." Do this for 10 minutes, using a timer if necessary.

There are numerous other relaxation techniques, including meditation, autohypnosis, progressive relaxation, and biofeedback. Consider using one to give yourself an instant vacation. You'll discover the benefits far outweigh the small loss of time.

193 Soar with your strengths

"Find out what you do well—and do more of it. Find out what you don't do well—and stop doing it." That recommendation comes from the book *Soar with Your Strengths*, by Donald O. Clifton, Ph.D., and Paula Nelson (Dell, 1995).

Strengths, the authors say, are things you do well and learn easily that produce a high degree of satisfaction and pride and generate psychological and/or financial rewards. Weaknesses are those things you don't do well and at which you don't significantly improve even after repeated tries. They intrude on your productivity and self-esteem and cause undue stress. No matter how dedicated you may be to improving yourself, the authors say, you'll never transform weaknesses into strengths.

ACTION STEP

The goal is to concentrate on your strengths and manage your weaknesses. One technique: Delegate tasks you don't do well or enjoy to those whose strengths lie in these areas. Then, use your time for more constructive pursuits.

"I struggled for a while with the hiring, management, and occasional firing of employees in our office," an Illinois O.D. admitted, "but I wasn't good at it and didn't like the job. One of my partners, much better suited for these matters, took over—and everyone's happier, employees included."

Some of the happiest optometrists I know are those who have concentrated their efforts on what they do well and enjoy doing.

Identifying weaknesses and emphasizing strengths in yourself and others is one of the most valuable and liberating discoveries you can make. It's also the surest route to achieving a high-performance optometric practice.

REALITY CHECK

"We doctors have a tendency to think we do everything best," says James K. Kirchner, O.D., Lincoln, NE. "Not so. We should do the things that only we can do, and train our staff to do the rest."[1]

194 Add a sense of fun to your practice

By making work enjoyable, says consultant Matt Weinstein, Ph.D., you help create the kind of organization to which your employees will want to make a long-term commitment and where turnover and burnout will be minimal. The intentional use of fun, he adds, can have an enormous impact on team building, stress management, employee morale, and the way patients are treated.[2]

Does this sound appealing? From the success files of high-performance practices, here are some ideas to generate a sense of fun in an office:

- Let people bring homegrown, homemade, or store-bought food to work on a rotating basis. Snack food is fun and promotes camaraderie. Establish a budget for the purpose.
- Even better, contract with a local produce distributor to supply your office with fresh fruit when in season. A fruit snack is a healthy treat and an energy-boosting alternative to coffee break

foods. Start with once a week to see how it goes. An added benefit: It will make employees feel they are special and they work in a special place.

- Place a dry-erase board in a central location where anyone (doctors or staff members) can write a compliment or thank you to anyone else.
- Have in-office lunches, catered or otherwise. These are great for staff meetings, celebrations, and bad-weather days.
- Fresh flowers, from a garden or delivered by a florist, are always uplifting and well worth the investment.
- Have parties, celebrations, and plenty of public pats on the back for achieving practice goals, employee birthdays, anniversaries, going away or "welcome aboard" occasions, or perhaps for no reason at all. Exchange gag gifts.
- Have a staff lounge where employees can take a break, renew their spirits, have a snack or a group luncheon, or simply let their hair down. Decorate with humorous posters, cartoons, anti-stress toys. A microwave oven is a must. Exercise equipment is another option.

You don't have to be elaborate. Fun activities need only provide a change of pace, a way to unwind if only for a few minutes, a way to celebrate and appreciate each other.

The mood of a practice is important. If your practice is an upbeat place to be, your patients will pick up on it, and you and your staff will be better for it.

At the Long Beach, NY, office of South Nassau Dermatology, a sign at the receptionist's desk had everyone chuckling:

> *If You Are Grouchy, Irritable, or Just Plain Mean, There Will Be a $10 Charge for Putting Up with You*

195 Emotional economics

I am indebted to Harriette and Bill Carney, D.V.M., in Meridian, MS, for the provocative phrase, *emotional economics*. It refers to the dilemma of whether it's worth the time, money, and stress to deal with the handful of patients who are unreasonable, demanding, and/or unappreciative of you and your staff's best efforts. An example is the kind of patient who is forever complaining—and whom there is no pleasing.

There are basically two solutions to this dilemma: If the economic benefits are worth it and/or the emotional costs are tolerable, then grin and bear it. If not, consider *dismissing* the patient, being as nice as you can about it.

"The doctor-patient relationship can be terminated in a variety of ways," writes John G. Classé, O.D., J.D., "but the most common is completion of treatment, which renders the continuation of the relationship unnecessary. The doctor is also free to withdraw from a case for any reason satisfactory to himself, including failure of the patient to pay for services or materials or to follow proper instructions, but there is the specter of abandonment under such circumstances.

"If a doctor wishes to withdraw from a case in which further care is required, it is advisable to notify the patient in writing and to retain a copy of the letter in the patient's record."[3]

The following is a sample letter suggested by Dr. Classé when withdrawing from the care of patient who requires further treatment:

Dear Mr./Mrs._____,
This letter is to inform you that I find it necessary to withdraw from the performance of further professional duties in your case because _____.

 Because you are still in need of treatment, I suggest you place yourself under the care of another practitioner without delay. If you are unable to obtain necessary services, I will continue to provide care for a reasonable period not to exceed _____. When you determine who your provider will be, with your consent I will make available to this practitioner the case history and other information concerning the diagnosis and treatment you have received from me.
 Sincerely,

_____ , O.D.

Optometrists who have taken this step tell me they get a variety of actions. Some of the complainers realize they've been out of line, apologize for their behavior, and become model patients; others take the hint and leave.

As a speaker, I've asked countless audiences of optometrists and staff members if anyone has ever *regretted* dismissing patients who couldn't be pleased. The only regret I've heard (and it's expressed frequently) is "I wish we had done it *sooner*."

REALITY CHECK

Lawyers advise that you should check with your malpractice insurer before taking any steps related to dismissing a patient. There are important issues regarding abandonment that need to be considered, including those that exist within the confines of a managed-care plan's provider panel.

196   Unrealistic expectations

Perhaps the saddest mistake of practice management, one that causes endless frustration and stress, is having *unrealistic expectations*. Here are some of the more common expectations that create a blueprint for disappointment and stress.

• You Can Find or Develop the "Perfect" Employee

Reality Check.   Do you expect your employees to be as dedicated, hard-working, energetic, and vitally interested in your patients and the success of your practice as you are? High expectations are fine. Studies show that employees tend to live up to their employers' expectations; it's called the *Pygmalion effect*. But *unrealistic expectations* are, by definition, unattainable.

If you have unrealistic expectations about employees, you'll be frustrated by what you perceive as unmotivated employees. They'll forever disappoint you.

Your employees, in turn, will be frustrated because it will seem as if nothing they do will be good enough to earn your approval and appreciation.

The result? Resentment and stress—on both sides.

Solution. Your expectations of employees may be unrealistic. You may not have hired the right people for your practice or have them doing the things they do best or *like* doing. On the other hand, it may be your management style that's at fault. An employee survey may pinpoint the problem (see Chapter 11).

- Your Partners and Associates Should Work as Hard as You Do

If you're frustrated by partners or associates who lack your motivation, remember that the drive to achieve is not uniformly distributed. Your style may be to keep pushing for higher and higher revenues, no matter what it takes to achieve them. When you arrive at some predetermined benchmark, it probably also seems perfectly natural to push on to a new and even higher goal.

When you look back, however, you may find your partners or associates lagging behind and making no special effort to keep up with you. One explanation: They may not have the drive to "climb the mountain because it's there." Some may be content to relax in the meadow part-way up, or pursue other goals such as spending more time with their families, sailing, whatever. In fact, they may think you are as strange as you think they are.

Reality Check. Problems often arise because of the presumption by one person that the other person will cooperate in a plan that has never actually been discussed between the two. The fact is they may have very different agendas.

- You Can Change Other People

Reality Check. Do you believe that if you are persuasive and persistent enough, you can change, *really change* another person? Do you think, for example, you can change an associate's mindset about continuing education or buying new equipment? Or get a partner to work harder, faster, or take more of an entrepreneurial interest in the practice? Trying to change other people's beliefs to conform to yours assumes their priorities and motivations are the same as yours. That's possible, but unlikely.

Solution. Accept that you can change people—but not very much. There are several alternatives: One is to keep trying but, perhaps, with a different approach. Another is to negotiate your differences;

reach a win/win compromise. If necessary, adopt a "what is, is" phi-losophy and learn to live with the situation. Severing the relationship is another option if you're in a position to do it.

After a recent seminar, an optometrist wrote me: "When I returned to the office, I split with my partner of 13 years. It was the hardest but best thing I ever did."

- You Can Please Every Patient, Every Time

Reality Check. Do you believe that you can please every patient who comes to your office? Do you take it personally when you don't or can't? The fact is some patients are impossible to please and drift from one practice to another, yours included. Others are more cost-conscious or demanding than your office policies allow.

Solution. Unless the numbers are getting out of hand, don't be too hard on yourself over lost patients. Turnover goes with the territory.

Take the advice of the late movie mogul, Louis B. Mayer: "I can't tell you the formula for success," he said. "But I can tell you the formula for *failure*: Try to please everyone."

BOTTOM LINE

As the poet said, a man's reach should exceed his grasp. Have goals that are realistic and attainable and with which you are com-fortable. Most importantly, have expectations that enable you to enjoy your patients, colleagues, staff, and your own impressive achievements.

197 Power of reframing

When I finally quit smoking many years ago, I considered it one of the hardest yet most rewarding things I've ever done. I had previously tried to quit, several times in fact, but found it difficult and resumed smoking. The problem was that I viewed quitting as a *deprivation* of something I enjoyed. I rationalized that life is too short and too stress-ful to torture myself.

What finally enabled me to quit once and for all was viewing the process not as a *deprivation*, but rather as a *gift* to my family and myself; a gift that is estimated to be a staggering *two minutes per cigarette!* This thought reinforced my resolve, sustained my motivation, and made quitting a *positive* act rather than a negative one.

Psychologists call this process reframing—it transforms the meaning of a situation and your response to it. For example, many people believe that the "butterflies in the stomach" associated with public speaking are bad, a sign of nervousness and inadequacy. They can, however, reframe their thoughts about such butterflies by viewing this anxiety as a positive source of energy that adds extra zest to their performance. It's worked for me. After more than 2,500 speaking engagements, I still get butterflies before a presentation, but it pumps me up and improves my delivery. The trick is to teach those butterflies to fly in formation.

There are countless situations that arise in optometric practice that are often viewed in a negative way. Examples include managed care, no-shows, evening hours, telephone shoppers, patient complaints, refunds, and staff turnover. Yet each of these has a component that could be viewed as an *opportunity* to differentiate your practice, exceed patient expectations, improve the image of your practice, or generate practice growth—*if* you choose to focus on the *positive* aspects rather than the negative.

ACTION STEP

Reframing is a powerful strategy for coping with stressful situations. Use it professionally or personally to change the polarity of your thinking from "negative" to "positive."

It may be the best gift you ever give yourself.

198 Not to decide is to decide

Practice management decisions are seldom easy. Invariably, there are arguments both for and against almost any course of action, such as the following:

- Raising your fees
- Hiring an associate
- Breaking up a partnership that's gone sour
- Buying a building
- Buying new equipment
- Adding an in-office lab
- Developing a subspecialty
- Trying to successfully combine career and family
- And on and on . . .

Most optometrists I've interviewed rely on four methods of decision making in dealing with such matters:

1. *Conformity.* When it comes to fees and hours, many optometrists check around, see what others are doing, and then follow suit. Conformity is easy, but it stifles practice growth. I've seen practitioners worry that if they're the first to raise fees or shorten their hours, patients will leave in droves. But, when the big day comes, patients take such changes in stride, and it's often their colleagues who then follow suit.

2. *Habit.* Some O.D.s adopt "we've done well without it until now"–type thinking. The problem is that the marketplace has changed and become more competitive. Patients have higher expectations. Your basic services and out-of-date equipment have served you well; it's time for change. Bernard Marcus, CEO of Home Depot, summed it up well when he said, "In today's highly competitive environment, the sure path to oblivion is to stay exactly where you are."

3. *Default.* Unable to decide whether to raise fees, buy new equipment, hire a new associate, or perhaps fire someone who has become more of an irritant than an asset to the practice, some optometrists do nothing: That's management by default, and the problems continue. Not to decide is to decide.

4. *Conscious decision.* It's sitting down, weighing the pros and cons, and making a decision. Few management decisions offer a clear choice, 100% one way or the other or even 80/20 or 60/40. Most decisions are of the 55/45 type or, tougher yet, 51/49.

One solution: Make two columns of advantages and disadvantages of a given course of action. Then base your decision on whichever column is longest or most compelling.

A second solution: If you find your thinking is polarized by either/or alternatives, consider a third option by visualizing a continuum, in which one choice is at one end and the other choice is at the other end. Then, visualize a place along the continuum that offers a third choice: a compromise alternative. For example, instead of buying (or not buying) a new piece of equipment, consider leasing it. Instead of deciding to take in a partner (or continue in solo practice), consider hiring a part-time, salaried associate to see how it goes.

REALITY CHECK

Most management decisions can be reversed if necessary. The feedback I often get about management decisions that were endlessly deliberated and finally made is "I wish I had done this 5 years sooner!"

FROM THE SUCCESS FILES

"If you never take risks, you will never be successful," says Walter S. Ramsey, O.D., F.A.A.O., Charleston, WV. "One risk I took was to invest more than $1.5 million in a new office building. I bought property in a developing area of town and committed to constructing a 7,000-square-foot state-of-the-art building. I could have taken the money and built a condo in Florida, but I decided to put it back into my practice. Few investments will pay off more substantially than your practice. But you have to be willing to take risks."[4]

---

199 Will you have regrets?

Throughout the years, I've asked countless optometrists, "Looking back, what's been the biggest regret in managing your practice?" The following are among the most frequent answers.

• I Didn't Spend More Time with My Family

Many optometrists promise their families: "Not now—later." It results in much borrowing against the future. The assumption? There will always be a future. Time slips by, however—and is gone.

You probably know at least one parent who laments the loss of children for whom he or she never had time, and who are now grown and gone. I recall one optometrist who, in his acceptance speech for his state association's "Optometrist of the Year" plaque, lamented the fact that he had devoted so much time to his profession that his children never fully knew him.

An Illinois optometrist was torn between having evening hours and being at home with his family. After much deliberation, he put a sign in his reception area that read: "Starting January lst, Daddy's office will close at 6:00 p.m." It was signed, "Debbie and Billy." He lost very few patients.

• I Didn't Move Sooner to an Entirely New Location

Despite the loss of major industry in the area and declining economic conditions, these optometrists kept postponing a move to a more favorable location, hoping the problems would go away. Once the move was made, most of those with whom I've spoken agree that their second practice is bigger, better, and less stressful than the first, and the time it took to get it there was much less than anticipated.

"I learned the hard way," says Robert A. Koetting, O.D., F.A.A.O., St. Louis, MO, "that higher rent for the right location is a good investment. When I moved into a high-rise office building in an upscale neighborhood, the practice boomed. I realized afterward that I should've done it sooner."[5]

• I Didn't Remodel/Redecorate My Office Sooner

The optometrists who have this regret admit, "I never realized how bad it was until we redecorated and everyone told us how nice it was—and what an *improvement* it was."

• I Didn't Raise My Fees Sooner

Those who say this agree that the complaints they got about higher fees were not nearly as numerous as they had feared. Most patients take reasonable, periodic fee increases in stride. Many don't even notice. Even those optometrists who lost patients owing to fee increases reported an improved overall profitability. Sometimes, less is more.

200 Carpe diem!

At Cornell University, psychologists Thomas Gilovich and Victoria Husted Medvec asked nursing home residents, Cornell students, employees, and professors emeritus to describe the biggest regrets of their lives. Using questionnaires, phone surveys, and one-on-one interviews, they obtained 230 responses.

The results indicate that what those surveyed most regret are the things in life they *failed to do*, not the things they did—by a margin of nearly 2 to 1! The most commonly listed regrets? Missed educational opportunities and failures to "seize the moment."[6]

ACTION STEPS

What if all possibilities were open to you? If money were no object, what's the first thing you would do?

A Vancouver, British Columbia practitioner took a 6-month leave of absence from his group practice. He traveled with his wife and two children to the South Pacific: Tahiti, the Cook Islands, and New Zealand. It took some rearranging of priorities to do it but resulted in a once-in-a-lifetime adventure. His assessment of the experience? "You don't just have a recharged battery," he told me. "You have a whole new motor."

201 Hard-learned lessons about stress and other things that go bump in the night

- No one has ever said on his or her deathbed, "I wish I had spent more time at the office."
- A bad partner is worse than no partner.
- In most cases, the things that happen in practice are never as good or as bad as they seem at the time.
- Striving for perfection is a blueprint for high-stress living.

- An optometrist, being honest with himself, told me: "Optometry didn't cause my mid-life crisis. I did."
- It's not what happens to us, but rather, our *perceptions* of what happens to us, that causes almost all forms of emotional stress.
- Robert S. Elliot, M.D., put it best in his "Rules to live by: (1) Don't sweat the small stuff. (2) It's all small stuff."
- David Cook, O.D., author of *When a Child Struggles*, has written, "While you must do only that with which you are comfortable, that with which you are comfortable may change over time."
- For every minute you are angry, you lose 1 minute of happiness.
- Psychologists say the key to enjoying your work is an old, nearly forgotten principle: Do your best, not just for the patient but for yourself.
- Susan Gromacki, O.D., lecturer in ophthalmology, University of Michigan Medical School, Ann Arbor, MI, said, "We have so many options for women to combine family life with a career in optometry. Each woman must decide what works best for her. None of these choices is wrong."
- Rudy Engholm, J.D., told me, "Seventy-five percent of my clients could have avoided lawsuits if someone had simply said, 'I'm sorry.'"
- The definition of insanity is doing the same thing again and again— and expecting different results.
- Recognize that younger and older doctors have had very different training and often, different attitudes about why they have chosen optometry, how they want to practice, and what they hope to get out of it. The only way to bridge that gap is constant and open communication.
- Mihaly Csikszentmihalyi, University of Chicago psychology researcher and author of *Flow: The Psychology of Optimal Experience*, said "Make a list of the things that are important in your life, then the things you spend most of your time doing. Cut back on the activities that don't match up with what truly matters to you, things that you've outgrown or are doing only out of obligation."
- The greatest risk is not taking one.
- "Nothing will ever be attempted if first, every possible objection must be overcome" (posted in the boardroom of one of America's largest corporations).

In the spirit of "exceeding expectations," here's one-more-than-promised secret of a high-performance optometric practice.

202 A memory jogger for overlooked tasks

When was the last time you did any of the following?

- Congratulated a staff member for a "job well done"
- Gave a staff member a raise without being asked
- Updated your business office
- Repainted, wallpapered, or redecorated your office
- Brought job descriptions up-to-date
- Conducted performance reviews
- Approached your staff about "job enrichment"
- Had your receptionist telephone patients who are overdue for an examination to see if they are aware of the time lapse and would like to make an appointment
- Raised your fees
- Reviewed the long-range plans for your practice
- Purchased new equipment for your office
- Had a lively, give-and-take staff meeting
- Attended a practice management seminar with your staff
- Determined if low-paying managed-care plans are covering your chair costs
- Asked patients for feedback about the quality of care and service they received in your office
- Asked your staff for their insights and ideas about practice-related issues
- Visited a successful colleague's office
- Saw your child/children in a school play, sports event, or related activity
- Wrote a note of thanks to an optical laboratory, a manufacturer or distributor, an officer of your association, or an ophthalmic journal
- Told your staff how important they are to your practice and how much you appreciate them

If these questions have jogged you into action, then they have served their purpose.

Notes

1. Kirchner JK. Start Practicing for the Future Today. *Optometric Management*, July 2000, 11S–14S.
2. Weinstein M. *Managing to Have Fun at Work*. New York: Simon & Schuster, 1996.
3. Classé JG. *Legal Aspects of Optometry*. Boston: Butterworth–Heinemann, 1989.
4. Ramsey WS. Extending Your Reach. *Optometric Management*, September 2001, 12–13.
5. Koetting RA. Unlocking Your Potential. *Optometric Management*, February 2001, 120.
6. Vital Signs. *Hippocrates*, January 1995, 16–17.

Epilogue

In This Special Moment of Life

The prologue to this book was a wake-up call. The epilogue is intended for quiet reflection.

The following paragraph is taken from a newsletter published by the Interfaith Nutrition Network of Glen Cove, NY, which helps hungry and homeless people.

Think freely. Practice patience. Smile often. Savor special moments. Make new friends. Rediscover old ones. Tell those you love that you do. Feel deeply. Forget trouble. Forgive an enemy. Hope. Grow. Be crazy. Count your blessings. Observe miracles. Let them happen. Discard worry. Give. Give in. Trust enough to take. Pick some flowers. Share them. Keep a promise. Look for rainbows. Gaze at stars. See beauty everywhere. Work hard. Be wise. Try to understand. Take time for people. Make time for yourself. Laugh heartily. Spread joy. Take a chance. Reach out. Let someone in. Try something new. Slow down. Be soft sometimes. Believe in yourself. Trust others. See a sunrise. Listen to rain. Reminisce. Cry when you need to. Trust life. Have faith. Enjoy wonder. Comfort a friend. Have good ideas. Make some mistakes. Learn from them. Celebrate life.

Appendix

Recording for the Blind and Dyslexic

Recording for the Blind and Dyslexic (RFB&D), a national nonprofit volunteer service organization, is the nation's largest educational library serving people who cannot effectively read standard print because of a visual impairment, dyslexia, or other physical disability. RFB&D has more than 90,000 titles on tape and compact disc in its Master Library, ranging from *Dr. Seuss* to *Introduction to Biology* to *Quantum Physics* and *Black's Law Dictionary*.

As a long-time volunteer reader for RFB&D, I wanted to include information about this organization, should it be of interest to someone you know. It also offers a wonderful opportunity for personal fulfillment, should you wish to become involved as a volunteer or donor.

Recording for the Blind, as it was originally known, was founded in 1948 to provide educational textbooks to blind World War II veterans who wanted to attend college under the GI Bill of Rights. Since that time, RFB&D's membership, programs, and services have expanded and diversified. In 2001, a quarter of a million books were circulated among RFB&D's 102,000 members in kindergarten through graduate school and beyond who are *learning through listening*.

"RFB&D's recorded textbooks have helped many students improve their reading skills while enabling some students to be mainstreamed into regular classrooms," says Gloria Safra, a teacher at the Anne Frank School in Philadelphia, PA. "Additionally, RFB&D has helped their self-esteem, which will provide a valuable foundation for their future."[1]

Jeffrey Lawler, a blind student at the Western University of Health Sciences College of Osteopathic Medicine of the Pacific in Pomona, CA,

---

1. Recording for the Blind and Dyslexic 2000 Annual Report.

praises the work of RBD&D. "It's been wonderful," he says, "a huge help to learning."[2]

At the heart of RFB&D's services are its 5,400 skilled and dedicated volunteers who record textbooks and provide other valuable services in their 32 facilities nationwide. Readers who are proficient in mathematics, science, finance, accounting, computer science, or other technical areas are needed to meet the increasing demands for materials in these subjects. RFB&D also needs volunteers for a variety of nonreading positions.

For further information or to become an RFB&D volunteer or donor, call toll-free, 866-RFBD-585, or visit their Web site at http://www.rbd.org.

---

2. Member Profile, published by Reading for the Blind and Dyslexic.

About the Author

As president of Success Dynamics Inc., Bob Levoy has conducted more than 2,500 seminars for a wide range of businesses and professional groups throughout North America and overseas. Among them have been countless optometric associations and conferences.

Bob holds three college degrees in marketing and optometry. He is the author of five books, numerous audiocassette albums, and more than 300 articles for business and professional journals, including *Optometric Management* for which he currently serves as a member of the Editorial Board and monthly columnist.

His unique background in the ophthalmic industry and health care professions has focused on market research and the development of programs to improve the performance and profitability of professional practices.

For information about his availability as a speaker, contact Bob Levoy at (516) 626-1353 or b.levoy@att.net.

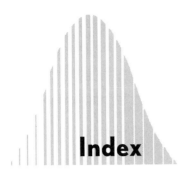

Index